Physiology for Therapeutic and Rehabilitation Practices

Current Approaches

Physiology for Therapeutic and Rehabilitation Practices

Current Approaches

Editor

G.L. Khanna

Narosa Publishing House

New Delhi   Chennai   Mumbai   Kolkata

Physiology for Therapeutic and Rehabilitation Practices
Current Approaches
164 pgs | 29 figs | 12 tbs

Editor

G.L. Khanna
Dean, Health Sciences
Faridabad Institute of Technology
Manav Rachna Educational Institutions
Sector 43, Delhi-Surajkund Road
Faridabad, India

NAROSA PUBLISHING HOUSE PVT. LTD.

22 Delhi Medical Association Road, Daryaganj, New Delhi 110 002
35-36 Greams Road, Thousand Lights, Chennai 600 006
306 Shiv Centre, D.B.C. Sector 17, K.U. Bazar P.O., Navi Mumbai 400 703
2F-2G Shivam Chambers, 53 Syed Amir Ali Avenue, Kolkata 700 019

www.narosa.com

ISBN 978-81-7319-920-2

Published by N.K. Mehra for Narosa Publishing House,
22 Delhi Medical Association Road, Daryaganj, New Delhi 110 002

Printed in India

Foreword

Manav Rachna Educational Institutions (MREI) and physiological Society of India (PSI) endeavored to conclude an appreciable task in bringing this book on "Current Approach of Physiology to Therapeutics and Rehabilitation". This publication attaches great significance in all respects particularly the application of latest research: innovations and emerging technologies that have taken place in the recent past. The application of this knowledge would certainly pave the way in a large scale for the benefit of society and mankind.

Renowned scholars, speakers from the University of Chicago, Boston University, Tulane University, University of Minnesota, University Sains Malaysia, Aga Khan University, Calcutta University, Vidyasagar University have made very valuable contribution.

Authors have taken sustained efforts to ensure that their contributions should reach the hands of many other research institutions, scientific bodies and educational institutions that are especially dedicated in similar research work. These articles provide in-depth study on neurophysiology, sport science, ergonomics, cardio respiratory, physiotherapy, nutrition, biochemistry, immunology and on environmental education.

The format, structure and content have been meticulously formulated with chapters by multidisciplinary team of authors who have made significant contribution in the field of physiology. They have emphasized the recent trends in clinical application of physiology in therapeutics and rehabilitation.

This book provides the core and concise knowledge of physiology keeping pace with the latest information and newer understanding of the discipline. Applied physiology and clinical correlation of physiology have been especially emphasized which can be taken as a base of research by scholars, that demands the integration of research evidence into practice rather that unquestioning acceptance of treatment formulae.

While I like to express my profound appreciation to all the authors and editorial board. I hope that this book stimulates the new generation of readers to take this fascinating specialty forward.

New Delhi

Dr. W. Selwamurthy
Distinguished Scientist & Chief Controller R&D
Government of India
Ministry of Defence
Defence Research and Development Organisation
201, DRDO Bhawan, New Delhi – 110011

Foreword

You have in your hands a compendium of papers contributed by renowned scientists from all parts of world on Current Approaches of Physiology to Therapeutics and Rehabilitation, jointly organized by Physiological Society of India (PSI) and Faridabad Institute of Technology (FIT), an organ of Manav Rachna Educational Institutions. This collection is a testimonial to the academic and professional commitment of the contributors. My sincere thanks and best wishes to them.

I am confident that the research findings and experiences shared by the experts from Asia, North America, Europe and Africa will add to the body of domain of knowledge and benefit the community of students, teachers, researchers, practitioners and experts alike.

Dr. O.P. Bhalla
President
Manav Rachna Educational Institutions (MREI)
Faridabad, Haryana, India

Preface

Physiology is a basic science to medicine, physiotherapy, nursing, health sciences, sports science and ergonomics. The concept of physiology is being refined at all levels to apply in these fields. Physicians, physiotherapists and heath professionals need to know the latest aspects of research and perfect techniques for application. This book is an attempt to fill some gap. Within this book you will find comprehensive articles on Neurophysiology, Sports science, Ergonomics, Cardio respiratory, Environmental aspect, Physiotherapy and Rehabilitation contributed by world renowned scientists from all over the globe. The latest researches in Physiology can be translated to application in Therapeutics and Rehabilitation Medicine. This book will be useful for Physiologists, Sports scientists, Therapists and Rehabilitation experts. I render my thanks to all the contributors for their articles for this book. I express my deep thanks to Dr. O.P Bhalla, Chairman, Manav Rachna Educational Institutions for his worthy guidance and constant support in bringing out this book. I am thankful to Col. (R) V.K Gaur, Executive Director for being a guiding force behind this book. I express my thanks to contributions made by all the faculty members of Department of Therapies and Health Sciences, Faridabad Institute of technology, Manav Rachna Educational Institute Faridabad.

G.L. Khanna

Contents

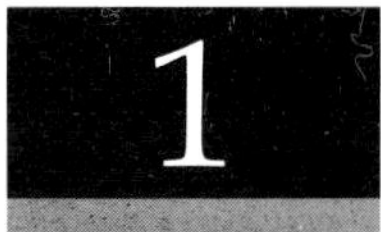

Cellular and Molecular Mechanism of Sleep-Dependent Memory Processing: Causal Interplay between Cellular Activation and Expression of Genes

Subimal Datta

Director, Sleep and Cognitive Neuroscience
Professor, Departments of Psychiatry and Behavioral Neurosciences
Boston University School of Medicine, 715 Albany Street, M-902, Massachusetts, USA

ABSTRACT

All animal species, from unicellular organisms to highly developed mammals, depend on their memory for survival. From the beginning of Vedic civilization until the early part of the twentieth century, many poets and philosophers have pondered the function of sleep and dreaming. These thinkers came to a common conclusion that one of the most important functions of sleep is to nurture memory. Most of these early philosophers believed that memory traces are subject to a time-dependent decay process. During this process, the decay rate is believed to be slower during sleep than wakefulness. Thus, memory benefits following a period of sleep were a result of a lack of sensory interference during sleep. Over the last three decades, however, the beneficial effects of sleep in strengthening memory have been explained by the emergence of a new model, called the consolidation theory. According to this theory, sleep facilitates the consolidation process of new memories over time. Sleep and learning studies in both humans and animals, using a variety of protocols and test paradigms, have produced two different types of correlative evidence to support this consolidation theory: (i) learning training trials increase rapid eye movement (REM) sleep during the subsequent sleep period; (ii) post learning-training REM sleep deprivation impairs learning performance by impairing memory formation. This correlative evidence suggests that an organism homeostatically adjusts its REM sleep in response to memory consolidation demands. Despite this strong correlation between REM sleep and memory processing, only a handful of studies have been designed to elucidate the mechanisms involved in sleep-dependent memory processing. Our studies suggest that memory consolidation following learning requires processes selectively active during REM sleep. To explain part of this mechanism, this article reviews findings of recent studies that were designed specifically to explain how activation of the phasic pontine-wave (P-wave) generator is involved in memory processing during the post-training REM sleep period.

INTRODUCTION

Sleep is a highly evolved global behavioral state in the mammalian species. Sleep is not a homogenous state, rather a continuum of a number of mixed states. The different components of this sleep continuum in the mammalian species could broadly be divided into two major states: non-rapid eye movement (NREM) and rapid eye movement (REM). Over the last 50 years, phenomenological and mechanistic aspects of sleep have been studied more carefully and extensively than the waking states (reviewed in Datta and MacLean, 2007). We spend so much of our lives asleep, and the motivation of sleep is so powerful, it must have some very important physiological function. At its most basic level, the function of mammalian sleep can best be described as a restorative process of the brain and body. Recently, however, progressive research has revealed a host of vital functions to which sleep is essential. This article is intended to provide a brief overview of my lecture on the mechanism of sleep-dependent memory processing.

"We as a mammalian species, unconditionally surrender to sleep for almost one third of our life. Whenever someone thinks of sleep, the first thing that comes to his or her mind is "rest", while some others think of it as a waste of time. Sleep is not simply the absence of wakefulness or a state of rest — rather sleep is a dynamic behavior — Sleep is a special activity of the brain, controlled by the brain — by its specific mechanism, and the biggest beneficiary of sleep is the brain itself."

"Memory is the processes through which learned information is stored — Memory is a link with the past for future survival and service — Understanding how memories are stored in the brain is an essential step towards understanding ourselves."

REM SLEEP AND MEMORY FORMATION

Since the discovery of REM sleep, many animal studies of sleep and learning have focused on the role of REM sleep in memory consolidation (reviewed in Smith, 1985; Datta, 2006). Using a variety of protocols and test paradigms, sleep and learning studies in animals have demonstrated the following results: **(1)** Training of rats on both appetitive and aversive tasks, including multiple-goal maze, operant bar press, shuttle avoidance, and classical conditioning tasks, leads to an increase in subsequent REM sleep. These increases appear not to be due simply to the stress of the training protocol, but to active learning of new material. **(2)** The increased REM sleep often begins immediately after training and lasts for a limited period of time - a "REM sleep window". **(3)** REM sleep deprivation during these REM sleep windows, but not during earlier or later periods, can partially or even totally block improved task performance on subsequent retesting. Taken together, these animal studies suggest that memory consolidation following task training requires processes selectively active during REM sleep and that the organism homeostatically adjusts its REM sleep in response to memory consolidation demands. Like animal studies, many human studies of sleep and learning have also focused on REM sleep (reviewed in Smith, 1995; Maquet, 2001). Human studies have demonstrated that learning trials increase REM sleep in the subsequent sleep period. Some studies have looked at the effect of REM sleep deprivation on specific memory systems. In one study, REM sleep deprivation after training had no effect on declarative/explicit tasks such as word lists or paired associates and word recognition tasks, but hindered the subsequent performance of implicit/procedural tasks such as a word fragment completion task. Another study using a visual discrimination task also reported that REM sleep deprivation prevents improvement on procedural memory. Complementary to these REM sleep deprivation studies, one study compared the amount of learning on a declarative (paired associates) learning task and a procedural (mirror writing) task following periods of wake or sleep. It was found that NREM-rich sleep (i.e. the first half of the night) enhanced subsequent performance on the declarative memory task - but not the procedural task - compared with an equivalent amount of either NREM-poor sleep (i.e. the second half of the night) or wake time. In contrast, REM-rich sleep (during the second half of the night) enhanced performance on the procedural but not the declarative task. These results suggest that REM sleep plays a larger role in the consolidation of procedural memories while NREM sleep is more critical for declarative memory consolidation. More recently, another study using a procedural memory task (visual discrimination), demonstrated that the amount of overnight improvement was proportional to the amount of NREM sleep during the first quarter of the night, as well as to the amount of REM sleep in the last quarter.

Taken together, the combined animal and human studies support the concept that REM sleep contributes importantly to the process of memory consolidation, especially of a procedural learning task. The goal of this lecture is to present arguments and supporting data for the hypothesis that the activation of phasic pontine-wave (P-wave) generating cells in the brainstem is critical for sleep-dependent learning and memory processing. Since the focus of this lecture is on the P-wave, and it is most frequent during REM sleep, we will first briefly discuss the mechanisms for the generation and maintenance of REM sleep.

CELLULAR-MOLECULAR-NETWORK (CMN) MODEL OF REM SLEEP REGULATION

Sleep, especially REM sleep, provides an exceptional opportunity to study the brain based physical and physiological foundation of cognitive processes. As one proceeds from waking into NREM sleep and then REM sleep, a series of dramatic and well-defined changes occur in the neurophysiology and neurochemistry of the brain (reviewed in Datta & MacLean, 2007). REM sleep is characterized by a constellation of events including the following: **(1)** a desynchronized pattern of cortical EEG activity; **(2)** marked atonia of the postural muscles; **(3)** rapid eye movements; **(4)** a theta rhythm within the hippocampus; **(5)** field potentials in the pons (P-wave), lateral geniculate nucleus and occipital cortex [ponto-geniculo-occipital (PGO)] spikes; **(6)** myoclonic twitches, most apparent in the facial and distal limb musculature and **(7)** pronounced cardiorespiratory fluctuations.

According to the Cellular-Molecular-Network (CMN) model (Datta, 1995; Datta & MacLean, 2007), the individual events of REM sleep are generated by distinct cell groups located in the brainstem. They are discrete components of a widely distributed network rather than a single REM sleep "center." For example, muscle atonia is executed by the activation of neurons in the locus coeruleus alpha, rapid eye movements result from the activation of neurons in the peri-abducens reticular formation, hippocampal theta rhythm is produced via the activation of neurons in the pontis oralis, PGO waves emerge by the activation of neurons in the caudo-lateral peribrachial area of predator mammals and in the dorsal part of the nucleus subcoeruleus of prey mammals, muscle twitches appear with the activation of neurons in the nucleus gigantocellularis (especially the caudal part), and increased brain temperature and cardio-respiratory fluctuations occur via the activation of neurons in the parabrachial nucleus. The cortical EEG activation sign of REM sleep, however, is executed jointly by the activation of neurons in the mesencephalic reticular formation and rostrally-projecting bulbar reticular formation (also called medullary magnocellular nucleus). We would like to emphasize here that these particular cell groups are simply the executive neurons for an individual sign. For the final expression of an individual sign, the relevant executive neurons employ a specific neuronal circuit unique to that REM sleep sign. In essence, each of these REM sleep signs has a separate, specialized network. Thus, each of these REM sleep signs could be modulated with multiple neurotransmitters at multiple sites of their circuit.

Turn-on or turn-off conditions of REM sleep generating executive neurons are regulated by the ratio of available aminergic and cholinergic neurotransmitters within those cell groups. The source of aminergic neurotransmitters is the locus coeruleus (noradrenergic cells) and raphe nucleus (serotonergic cells), while cholinergic neurotransmitters originate from the laterodorsal tegmental and pedunculopontine tegmentum. The activity of both aminergic and cholinergic cells is approximately equal during wakefulness and the onset of NREM sleep results in an equal reduction in activity. Therefore, during wakefulness and NREM sleep the ratio of aminergic to cholinergic neurotransmitters in REM sleep generators is proportionate. During REM sleep, however, aminergic cell activities are markedly reduced or absent and cholinergic cell activities are comparatively high. The level of cholinergic cell activity during REM sleep is roughly thirty-five percent less than that of wakefulness. Thus, when a hypothetical ratio of aminergic and cholinergic neurotransmitters is 1:1, the REM sleep sign-generator remains in turned-off condition; however, when this ratio is 0:0.65, the generator is turned-on to express REM sleep signs (Datta & Siwek, 2002). For the detailed mechanisms of REM sleep generation, readers are referred to recent reviews (Datta, 1995; Datta and MacLean, 2007).

DESCRIPTION OF THE P-WAVE GENERATOR

Phasic activation of a group of neurons in the pontine tegmentum just prior to the onset of, and throughout REM sleep, generates a prominent field potential called the P-wave (Datta and Hobson, 1994, 1995; Datta et al., 1998). The P-wave is one of the most prominent physiologic signs of REM sleep. Since, in the cat, this potential originates in the pons (P) and propagates to the lateral geniculate body (G) and occipital cortex (O), it has been called the ponto-geniculo-occipital (PGO) wave (Datta, 1997). The P-wave in the rat is equivalent to the pontine component of the PGO wave in the cat (Datta et al., 1999). In the rat, this field potential is absent in the lateral geniculate body (LGB) due to the lack of afferent inputs from P-wave generating cells (Datta et al., 1998). Since this field potential is absent in the LGB of the rat, it is called the P-wave rather than PGO wave (Datta et al., 1999; Datta, 2000). This field potential has also been recorded from many other parts of the brain which receive excitatory inputs from the PGO-wave generation site (Datta, 1997). In addition to cats, the PGO wave has been documented and studied in other mammals including non-human primates, humans, and rodents (Datta, 1997). The P-wave is 75-150 mSec in duration and has amplitude of 100-150 μV. This wave occurs as a singlet and as clusters containing a variable number of P-waves (3-5 waves/burst) at a frequency range of 30-60 spikes/min during REM sleep (Datta, 1997, 2000). The P-wave generator in the cat and humans is located within the caudo-lateral part of the peribrachial area (Datta et al., 1992). In the rat, this P-wave generator is located within the dorsal part of the subcoeruleus nucleus (Datta et al., 1998).

Using specific monoclonal antibodies, P-wave generating cells have been identified as glutamatergic (Datta, 2006). Single cell recording studies have shown that these P-wave generating neurons discharge high-frequency (>500 Hz) spike bursts (3-5 spikes/burst) in the background of tonically increased firing rates (30-40 Hz) during the P-wave related states of tS-R (transitional state between NREM and REM sleep) and REM sleep (Datta & Hobson, 1994; Datta, 1997). Normally, these glutamatergic P-wave generating cells remain silent during W and NREM sleep. Neuroanatomical pathway tracing studies have demonstrated that functionally identified P-wave generator cells project to the hippocampus, amygdala, entorhinal cortex, visual cortex and many other regions of the brain known to be involved in cognitive processing (Datta et al., 1998). It has also been demonstrated that the dorsal hippocampus and amygdala receive direct anatomical projections from these P-wave generating cells. Activation of the P-wave generator increases glutamate release in the dorsal hippocampus and increases the frequency of hippocampal theta wave activity (Datta et al., 1998; Datta, 2006). In addition to glutamate release, activation of P-wave generating cells increases activation of plasticity-related gene and protein synthesis in the dorsal hippocampus and the amygdala (Saha & Datta, 2005; Ulloor & Datta, 2005; Datta, 2006).

MODEL OF SLEEP-DEPENDENT MEMORY CONSOLIDATION AND LONG TERM STORAGE

According to our model (for details see Datta and Patterson, 2003), during wakefulness, external information is randomly input into the brain and stored in the neocortex and other storage areas. This process is called acquisition of information. At the time of acquisition, a representational catalogue of temporarily stored information is created in the amygdala, hippocampus, and parahippocampal areas. At this stage, the short-term memories are labile and subject to disruption and/or loss. In order to become stable and permanent, these labile short-term memories move through a consolidation process

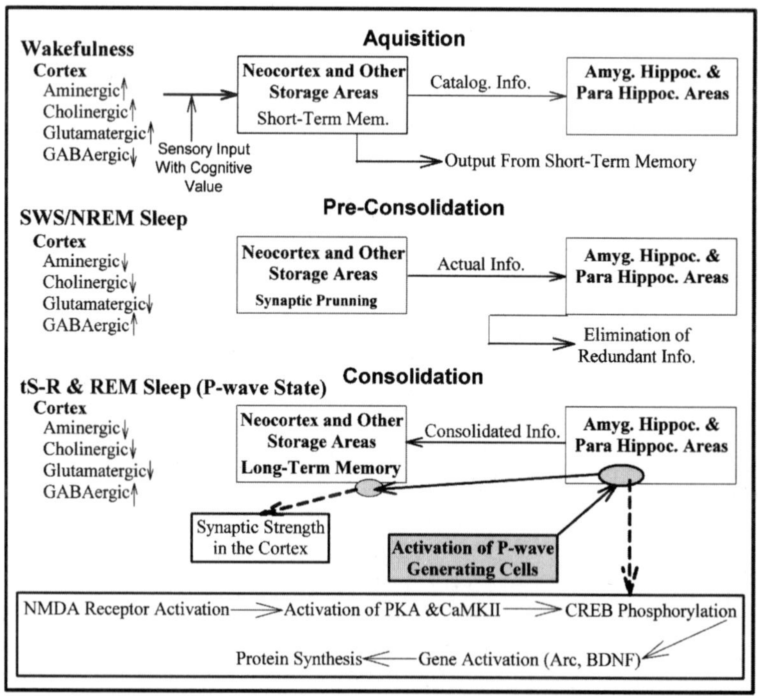

during the subsequent sleep period. During NREM sleep, the actual detailed information that had been temporarily stored in the neocortex and other storage areas is transferred to the amygdala, hippocampus, and parahippocampal areas. This is an important pre-consolidation phase. During this phase, some of the redundant information is eliminated to attenuate signal to noise ratio. During the P-wave related sleep states, the transition between NREM sleep and REM sleep, activation of P-wave generating cells in the pons reactivates the amygdala, hippocampus, and parahippocampal areas to organize the random information acquired during wakefulness. This process is called consolidation of information. Once information is consolidated, it is ready to be stored in the permanent storage. Theta-frequency waves generated during REM sleep help to bind that consolidated information into the long-term memory storage in the neocortex and other storage areas.

EVIDENCE TO LINK P-WAVE GENERATOR ACTIVATION WITH SLEEP-DEPENDENT MEMORY PROCESSING

Memory is a psychological function for which there are no direct methods of measurement. Memory can only be inferred from performance expressed at a behavioral level. Therefore, supporting arguments presented below are based only on the direct evidence that links neuronal activation of the P-wave generator to learned performance. Behavioral and physiological studies provide considerable evidence to support the idea that REM sleep is a highly favorable behavioral state for the consolidation and integration of memories (Datta & Patterson, 2003; Datta et al., 2004). Using two different types of learning paradigms, two-way active avoidance and spatial learning in the Morris water maze, we have shown that learning training increases REM sleep P-wave activity (Datta, 2000; 2006). More importantly, the results of these two studies have shown that the increase in P-wave density during the post-training REM sleep episodes is positively correlated with the effective consolidation, retention, and recall of the learning task. Together, the results of these two studies indicated that P-wave generator activation may have a positive influence in the REM sleep-dependent memory processing of two-way active avoidance and spatial navigational learning behavior. Based on the results of these two studies, we have tested a hypothesis that supplementary activation of the P-wave generator during REM sleep may enhance consolidation and integration of memories, resulting in improved learning (Mavanji & Datta, 2003). Indeed, the results of this study demonstrated that the supplemental activation of the P-wave generator above the normal post-training increase in P-wave activity boosts retention of learning in the test trials (Mavanji & Datta, 2003).

Animal and human studies of sleep and learning have demonstrated that REM sleep deprivation following learning training trials blocks the expected improvement in performance on subsequent testing. Based on the facts that the post-training REM sleep deprivation blocks improvement in memory performance and P-wave generator activation enhances memory consolidation, we have tested a hypothesis that the P-wave generator activation could eliminate the learning impairment produced by post-training REM sleep deprivation. Our results demonstrated that the activation of P-wave generator prevents REM sleep deprivation-induced learning impairment (Datta et al., 2004). The results of this study further substantiate the idea that activation of the P-wave generator during REM sleep enhances a physiological process of memory processing which naturally occurs during post-learning REM sleep. Based on this observation, we hypothesized that the elimination of P-wave generating cells would prevent memory processing and would ultimately attenuate retention and improvement of learning abilities in post-sleep test trials. The results from the post-lesion sleep recording sessions indicated that the lesions in the P-wave generator eliminated P-waves during REM sleep without changing the amounts of time spent in W, NREM sleep, or REM sleep. In these P-wave generator lesioned rats, acquisition of avoidance learning and post-training sleep-wake changes were identical to those of sham-lesioned rats. However, in the test trials, after undisturbed sleep-wake, P-wave generator lesioned rats had no retention of avoidance memory. These findings provided direct evidence that P-wave-generating cells are crucial for normal REM sleep-dependent memory processing. This evidence also supports the idea that the P-wave generator in the brainstem acts as an on-switch to provide activating input to forebrain structures for sleep-dependent memory processing.

As part of the REM sleep-dependent memory consolidation mechanism, physiological studies have suggested that the reactivation of the hippocampus, amygdala, and some specific parts of the cerebral cortex may be pre-requisite for off-line memory processing (Datta et al., 2005; Datta, 2006). Parallel to this behavioral and physiological research, cellular and molecular studies demonstrate that neuronal activation-dependent gene expression and protein synthesis in the hippocampus and amygdala are necessary for long-term neuronal plasticity and long-term memory formation (Saha & Datta, 2005; Ulloor & Datta, 2005). Neuronal activation-dependent gene expression and protein synthesis for long-term neuronal plasticity and memory formation require post-synaptic NMDA receptor activation. This NMDA receptor-mediated post-synaptic activation identifies a need for glutamatergic input to the hippocampus and amygdala. Similarly, it has also been suggested that, for REM sleep-dependent memory processing, reactivation in the hippocampus, amygdala, and cortex would require an active triggering input from the REM sleep sign generating cell groups (Datta 2000). It is known that REM sleep is generated by the simultaneous activation and inhibition of a distributed network in the pons and caudal midbrain (reviewed in Datta & MacLean, 2007). If neuronal reactivation is a prerequisite for memory processing then, what part(s) of the REM sleep generating network is involved in the neuronal activation-dependent memory processing? Based on four different types of evidence, we suggest that the P-wave generating cells of the

REM sleep generating network is involved in the neuronal activation-dependent memory processing. First, P-waves are generated by the phasic excitation of a group of glutamatergic cells located in the REM sleep sign-generating network in the pons (Datta & Hobson, 1994; Datta et al., 1998; Datta, 2006). Secondly, P-wave generating cells send their efferent projections to the hippocampus, amygdala, and other forebrain structures known to be involved in memory processing (Datta et al., 1998). The third, activation of P-wave generating cells increases plasticity-related gene activation and protein synthesis (Saha & Datta, 2005; Ulloor & Datta, 2005). Lastly, selective elimination of P-wave generating cells blocks this NMDA receptor activation-mediated memory processing in the dorsal hippocampus and amygdala (Mavanji et al., 2004; Datta et al., 2005).

SUMMARY AND CONCLUDING REMARKS

Here, I have discussed some of the compelling evidence that I believe to be significant for our understanding of mechanisms for REM sleep-dependent memory processing. These findings are the following: **(1)** Improvement of two-way active avoidance and Morris water maze spatial learning performance in the test trials session is proportional to the increase in phasic P-wave density during the REM sleep episodes after training trials (Datta, 2000; 2006). **(2)** After two-way active avoidance learning training trials, immediate supplemental activation of the P-wave generator above the normal post-training increase in P-wave activity significantly increases retention of learning in the test trials (Mavanji and Datta, 2003). **(3)** Activation of the P-wave generator prevents the two-way active avoidance memory impairing effects of post-training REM sleep deprivation (Datta et al., 2004). **(4)** Elimination of P-waves by selective elimination of P-wave generating cells prevents retention of two-way active avoidance learning in the test trials (Mavanji et al., 2004). **(5)** P-wave generating cells are glutamatergic, and activation of those cells releases glutamate from their axon terminals in the dorsal hippocampus (Datta, 2006). **(6)** Functionally identified P-wave generator cells project to the hippocampus, amygdala, entorhinal cortex, visual cortex and many other regions of the brain known to be involved in cognitive processing (Datta et al., 1998). **(7)** We have demonstrated that the P-wave generator activation-dependent memory processing of avoidance learning involves active interaction between the dorsal hippocampus and P-wave generator (Datta et al., 2005). **(8)** The memory processing of two-way active avoidance that requires activation of the P-wave generator also causes activation of the transcription factor CREB and simultaneous expression of Arc and BDNF genes in the dorsal hippocampus and amygdala (Datta & Saha, 2005; Ulloor & Datta, 2005). These findings are significant because they provide most direct evidence to substantiate the idea that P-wave generator activation during post-training REM sleep is critical for sleep-dependent memory processing of two-way active avoidance and spatial learning.

At present, our understanding of REM sleep-dependent memory processing mechanisms remains incomplete. Nevertheless, based on the existing findings, I suggest that learning training causes an increased homeostatic demand for the activation of P-wave generating cells in the brainstem that ultimately increases the total duration of P-wave related states, tS-R and REM sleep and REM sleep. Activation of P-wave generating cells during post-learning REM sleep provides a glutamatergic-activating stimulus to the hippocampus and amygdala leading to the physiological reactivation and neuronal activation-dependent gene expression and protein synthesis necessary for long-term neuronal plasticity and memory formation.

Acknowledgments

This work was supported by the National Institutes of Health (USA) research Grants: NS 34004 and MH 59839. I would like to thank Jessica L. Shea for her assistance in preparing this manuscript.

Bibliography

1. Datta S. (1995). Neuronal activity in the peribrachial area: Relationship to behavioral state control. Neurosci. Biobehav. Rev. 19:67-84.

2. Datta S. (1997). Cellular basis of pontine ponto-geniculo-occipital wave generation and modulation. Cell. Mol. Neurobiol. 17:341-365.

3. Datta S. (2000). Avoidance task training potentiates phasic pontine-wave density in the rat: a mechanism for sleep-dependent plasticity. J. Neurosci. 20:8607-8613.

4. Datta S. (2006). Activation of phasic pontine-wave generator: A mechanism for sleep-dependent memory processing. Sleep Biol. Rhyth. 4:16-26.

5. Datta S and Hobson JA. (1994). Neuronal activity in the caudolateral peribrachial pons: relationship to PGO waves and rapid eye movements. J. Neurophysiol. 71:95-109.

6. Datta S and Hobson JA. (1995) Suppression of ponto-geniculo-occipital waves by neurotoxic lesions of pontine caudo-lateral peribrachial cells. Neurosci. 67:703-712.

7. Datta S and MacLean RR. (2007). Neurobiological mechanisms for the regulation of mammalian sleep-wake behavior: Reinterpretation of historical evidence and inclusion of contemporary cellular and molecular evidence. Neurosci. Biobehav. Rev. 31:775-824.

8. Datta S and Patterson EH. (2003). Activation of phasic pontine-wave (P-wave): a mechanism of learning and memory processing. In: Maquet P, Smith C, Stickgold R, eds. *Sleep and Brain Plasticity*. New York: Oxford University Press, pp. 135-156.

9. Datta S, Calvo JM, Quattrochi JJ and Hobson JA. (1992) Cholinergic microstimulation of the peribrachial nucleus in the cat. I. Immediate and prolonged increases in ponto-geniculo-occipital waves. Arc. Ital. Biol. 130:263-284.

10. Datta S, Siwek DF, Patterson EH and Cipolloni PB. (1998). Localization of pontine PGO wave generation sites and their anatomical projections in the rat. Synapse 30:409-423.

11. Datta S, Patterson EH and Siwek DF. (1999). Brainstem afferents of the cholinoceptive pontine wave generation sites in the rat. Sleep Res. Online 2:79-82.

12. Datta S, Mavanji V, Ulloor J and Patterson EH. (2004). Activation of phasic pontine-wave generator prevents rapid eye movement sleep deprivation-induced learning impairment in the rat: a mechanism for sleep-dependent plasticity. J. Neurosci. 24:1416-1427.

13. Datta S, Saha S, Prutzman SL, Mullins OJ and Mavanji V. (2005). Pontine-wave generator activation-dependent memory processing of avoidance learning involves the dorsal hippocampus in the rat. J. Neurosci. Res. 80:727-737.

14. Maquet P. (2001). The role of sleep in learning and memory. Science 294:1048-1052.

15. Mavanji V and Datta S. (2003). Activation of the phasic pontine-wave generator enhances improvement of learning performance: a mechanism for sleep-dependent plasticity. Europ. J. Neurosci. 17:359-370.

16. Mavanji V, Ulloor J, Saha S and Datta S. (2004). Neurotoxic lesions of phasic pontine-wave generator cells impair retention of 2-way active avoidance memory. Sleep 27:1282-1292.

17. Saha S and Datta S. (2005). Two-way active avoidance training-specific increases in phosphorylated cAMP response element-binding protein in the dorsal hippocampus, amygdala, and hypothalamus. Europ. J. Neurosci. 21:3403-3414.

18. Smith C. (1985). Sleep states and learning: A review of the animal literature. Neurosci. Biobehav. Rev. 9:157-168.

19. Smith C. (1995). Sleep states and memory processes. Behav. Brain Res. 69:137-145.

20. Ulloor J and Datta S. (2005). Spatio-temporal activation of cyclic AMP response element-binding protein, activity-regulated cytoskeletal-associated protein and brain-derived nerve growth factor: a mechanism for pontine-wave generation activation-dependent two-way active-avoidance memory processing in the rat. J. Neurochem. 95:418-428.

2

Serotonin Receptor Subtypes and Sexual Receptivity in the Female Rat

Arif Siddiqui, Ambreen Niazi and Saeeda Shaharyar

Department of Biological & Biomedical Sciences, Aga Khan University, Stadium Road
Karachi-74800, Pakistan

ABSTRACT

5-Hydroxytryptamine (5-HT) regulates sexual behaviour in the female rat via a number of its receptors. To investigate, the role of $5HT_7$ receptor ovariectomised rats primed with 10ìg oestradiol benzoate(OB) followed at 48 hours by 0.5mg progesterone, which induced receptivity in approximately half the animals, were treated with three agonists all exerting effects via $5HT_{1A}$ and $5HT_7$ receptors; 5-hydroxytryptophan, 8-hydroxy-2-(di-n-propylamino)tetralin 1-Br (8-OH DPAT) and 5-carboxy-aminotryptamine (5-CT) in the presence or absence of selective $5HT_{1A}$ and $5HT_7$ antagonists: WAY 100135 and SB269970-A. Compared to non-receptive animals the three agonists in the receptive group inhibited lordosis which was prevented by both the selective $5HT_{1A}$ and $5HT_7$ antagonists. When given alone, both WAY 100135 and SB 269970-A increased the lordosis in the non-receptive rats indicating that endogenous 5-HT acting on $5HT_{1A}$ and $5HT_7$ receptors may have a tonic inhibitory effect on receptivity. A comparison of OB priming doses on the effect of serotoninergic agents showed that the higher OB doses attenuated the inhibitory effect of 8-OH DPAT and enhanced the stimulatory effect of WAY 100135, but did not affect the actions of 5-CT or SB269970-A. The interaction between oestradiol and 5-HT activity on sexual behaviour may therefore be selective to the $5HT_{1A}$ pathway. Moreover, 5-HT7 receptor activation appears to mediate an inhibitory effect on female sexual behaviour and this may be a physiological effect as the selective 5-HT7 antagonist, SB 269970-A exerts stimulatory effect on sexual behaviour.

INTRODUCTION

Lordosis is an essential reflex for reproduction in female rats and many other mammals. It is produced as a response to copulatory stimulation by the male

(Pfaff and Modianos, 1985). The reflex is regulated via gonadal hormone-dependent modulation of serotoninergic (5-HT) system (Ahlenius et al., 1986; Mendelson, 1992). Serotoninergic modulation of female rat lordosis behaviour is believed to include both facilitatory and inhibitory components located in the ventromedial hypothalamus (Aiello-Zaldivar et al., 1992; Uphouse et al., 1992; Maswood et al., 1997). The latter study also implicates interaction with multiple 5-HT receptors within the ventromedial nucleus (VMN) of the hypothalamus. At least three 5-HT receptor families are known to influence lordosis by modulating the estrogen sensitive receptive field of some sensory neurons in the perineal region and 5-HT neurons in the VMN (McCarthy and Becker, 2002). Activation of 5-HT_{1A} receptors within the VMN either by 8-OH DPAT or buspirone inhibits lordosis (Uphouse et al., 1991; 1992; Jackson and Etgen, 2001). The effect has been shown to be reversed by WAY 100 635 leading to enhanced lordosis behavior acutely in female rats with a low estrous states (Kishitake and Yamanouchi, 2003). In sexually receptive rats, a $5\text{-HT}_{2A/2C}$ receptor antagonist also inhibits lordosis (Uphouse et al., 1996) whereas $5\text{-HT}_{2A/2C}$ receptor agonists facilitate the behavior in non-sexually receptive females (Wolf et al., 1998). An appropriate steroidal milieu thus does seem a pre-requisite and play some role in 5-HT-dependent modulation of lordosis, although lordotic response requires steroid priming, the response may vary depending not only on the dose regimen of steroids but also the serotoninergic transmitter system involved.

$5\text{-HT}_{2A/2C}$ receptors have also been shown to facilitate lordosis (Wolf et al., 1998) but had no effect on LH release, but the 5-HT_2 receptor antagonist, ritanserin, antagonized the inhibitory effect of both 5-HT and 8-OH DPAT on LH release (Siddiqui et al., 2000). Nonetheless, the presence of 5-HT_7 receptors in the hypothalamus (Varnas et al., 2004) and their potential involvement in circadian rhythms (Lovenberg et al., 1993) makes them a likely candidate for regulation of steroid hormone release and lordosis behavior. Identification of another receptor subtype of 5-HT with affinity towards 5-HT_7 receptor subtype and with moderate affinity to 8-OH DPAT, which also has some $5\text{-HT}_{1A/7}$ affinity, prompted us to investigate the role of this receptor subtype in lordosis behaviour. The likelihood that this receptor is involved is based on the fact that 5HT_7 receptors are involved in the inhibitory effect of 5-HT on LH release (Siddiqui et al., 2004) which like sexual behaviour is a steroid-dependent function (McEwen and Parsons, 1982). In addition, although the intracellular pathways mediating the effects of 5HT_{1A} and 5HT_7 receptor activation are different and can be in opposition (Barnes and Sharpe, 1999), the two subtypes appear to have similar effects on a number of physiological functions including phase re-setting of the circadian rhythm in the suprachiasmatic nucleus (Sprouse et al., 2005), anxiety (Takeda et al., 2005), inhibition of LH release in vivo (Siddiqui et al., 2000; 2004) and stimulation of GnRH activity in vitro (Hery et al., 1997). They have opposing effects on other functions such as pro-nociceptive response (Rocha-Gonzalez et al., 2005), mood (Lucki et al., 1994; Hedlund et al., 2005) and regulation of REM sleep (Thomas et al., 2003; Harvey et al., 2004). Since 5HT_{1A} agonists have a marked inhibitory effect on female sexual behaviour (Gorzalka et al., 1990; Uphouse et al., 1991; Kishitake and Yamanouchi, 2003) it is possible that activation of the $5HT_7$ receptor may also affect sexual behaviour either in a similar or in an opposite manner to $5HT_{1A}$ activation.

The effect of three serotoninergic agonists, 5-hydroxytryptophan (5-HTP; this is converted to 5-HT once within the central nervous system; CNS), 8-hydroxy-2- (di-n-propylamino) tetralin1-Br (8-OH DPAT) and 5-carboxy-aminotryptamine (5-CT), on female sexual behaviour have been observed in the absence and presence of a selective $5HT_{1A}$ antagonist, WAY 100135 (Fletcher et al., 1993) or a selective $5HT_7$ antagonist, SB269970-A (Thomas et al., 2000).In order to reveal putative stimulatory or inhibitory effects, the treatments were tested on rats that were subdivided into two groups according to their level of receptivity after steroid priming and before treatment with the serotonergic agents. It is assumed that rats exhibiting a low level of receptivity (lordosis quotient <50%) would reveal possible stimulatory effects of the 5HT agonists,while rats with a higher lordosis quotient (>50%) would reveal any inhibitory effects. The three agonists are non-selective (Hoyer et al., 1994; Bonaventure et al., 2002).

There are a number of reports showing that in ovariectomised rats, increasing the dose of the priming oestradiol benzoate treatment and repetition of steroid priming before repeated tests for sexual behaviour can induce desensitization of the response to the $5HT_{1A/7}$ agonist, 8-OH DPAT (Jackson and Uphouse, 1996; 1998; Jackson and Etgen, 2001).

METHODOLOGY

Animals, Housing Conditions and Surgical Procedures

Female Wistar rats from litters born and raised in the animal housing facility at Aga Khan University were weaned at 25 days of age. The rats were housed in polycarbonate shoebox cages, four to five like-sex littermates per cage. The colony room was maintained at about 24°C on a 12 hr light-dark cycle with lights off at 6:00 p.m. Rat chow and water were available ad lib.

Female rats of 75-80 days of age (180-225 gm) were anaesthetized with pentobarbitone then bilaterally ovariectomized via bilateral lumbar incision. Immediately post-surgery, these females were housed exactly in a way, described above.

Steroids-priming

Following recovery, groups of rats (n = 100 – 120) were primed with 10 µg OB subcutaneously 50 hr before the experiment. Administration of OB alone exerts a negative feedback effect on LH release and induces relatively low levels of plasma LH. 48 hr after the OB and 2 hr before the experiment, this treatment stimulates the release of an LH surge with a peak concentration about 2-3.5 hr after the P (0.5 mg, subcutaneously), associated with enhanced sexual receptivity. Steroids were dissolved in 0.1 ml corn oil as solvent vehicle. Two hours after progesterone lordosis was monitored 15 min. prior to testing against 5-HT agents. Female rats belonging to the treatment regimen of OB followed by P, showing an LQ of >55 % were regarded as receptive rats (n = 85). It should be noted that rats bred at the Aga Khan University appear to be relatively insensitive to steroid priming. Ten and 25 µg OB followed by progesterone according to many reports in the literature normally induce full receptivity. Our rats treated with this regime tended to fall into two sub-groups exhibiting either 15-20% lordosis quotient (LQ) or 50-60 % LQ, which were designated as non-receptive and receptive, respectively.

Groups of animals received one of the following treatment by intra-peritoneal injection (i.p.), saline (1ml/kg), 5-hydroxytryptophan (5-HTP; 10mg/kg; Sigma Co Ltd. Poole, UK), 8-hydroxy-2-(di-n-propylamino) tetralin 1-Br (8-OH DPAT; 0.15mg/kg; RBI. Natick MA, USA) or 5-carboxyamidotryptamine (5-CT; 1mg/kg; Tocris Bioscience, MO., USA). These were given alone or in animals pre-treated i.p. with either saline (1ml/ kg) or the $5HT_{1A}$ antagonist WAY100135 (5mg/kg; Wyeth Research Centre, Taplow, Bucks, UK) or the $5HT_7$ antagonist SB 269970-A (1mg/kg; Tocris Bioscience MO. USA). All drugs were dissolved in 0.9% w/v saline.

Behavioral Testing Procedures

Behavioral testing involved presentation of a test female to a sexually active male rat in a cylindrical pyrex arena measuring 50 cm in height and 30 cm in diameter. Each experimental female remained with a single male for 10 min. and observed for pelvic thrusting as an index of lordosis. If a male would not mount, the female was placed in a different arena containing another male. A female's response to a mount was considered a lordosis response if some degree of concavity of the back was observed (Siddiqui et al, 2006).

Experimental Design

All rats were subjected to a 15 min test for sexual behaviour, 50 hours and 2 hours after the OB and P priming, respectively (Pre-injection test). They then received either saline or one of the serotoninergic antagonists, (WAY 100135 or SB 269970-A). Twenty min after SB 269970-A and 60 min after WAY 100135, the animals received either saline or one of the serotoninergic agonists, 5-HTP, 8-0H DPAT or 5-CT and 15 min later they were tested for a second time (Post-injection test).

Based on the LQ% of the pre-injection test, rats in each treatment group were sub-divided into Non-Receptive (NR; LQ% < 50%) or Receptive (R; LQ% > 50%) and the effect of the treatments on these two sub-groups were assessed separately. It was assumed that any putative inhibitory effect would be revealed in the R subgroup and any stimulatory effect in the NR subgroup.

Experiment 1: All rats receiving 10µg/rat OB plus 0.5mg/rat progesterone (s.c.) as the priming regime were tested (pre-injection) and then received either saline followed by the agonists or were pre-treated with the antagonists before administering the agonists The treated animals were then tested again (post-injection).

Experiment 2: Groups of rats received either 10 µg or 25 µg OB followed by 0.5mg progesterone. They were then tested for sexual receptivity followed by administration of 8-0H DPAT or 5-CT and tested again 15 minutes later. This procedure was repeated twice at 14 day intervals, the same rats receiving the same agonist each time.Thus the effect of three consecutive administrations of the priming regime and the agonists was observed

Statistical Analysis

Comparison of pre-injection and post-injection LQ %s were made by Students' paired 't' test. Comparison of groups receiving different OB priming doses three times at fortnightly intervals were assessed by 1-way Analyses of Variance (ANOVA) with Repeated Measures. In all cases $P < 0.05$ was considered statistically significant.

RESULTS

Experiment 1: The effect of 5-HTP, 8-0H DPAT and 5-CT and selective $5HT_{1A}$ and $5HT_7$ antagonists on female sexual behaviour

Ovariectomised rats primed with 10µg OB and 0.5mg progesterone were subdivided into receptive (LQ > 50%) and non-receptive (LQ < 50%) based on their pre-injection behavioural test. The effect of the three agonists, 5HTP, 8-0H DPAT, (predominantly a $5HT_{1A}$ agonist with some $5HT_7$ activity) and 5-CT (with a higher affinity than the other agonists for the $5HT_7$ receptor, but also exerting potent effects on the $5HT_{1A}$ receptor) were assessed by comparison of the results of the post-injection test for behaviour with the pre-injection test.

Table 1 shows that in the receptive animals,which should reveal putative inhibitory effects, all 3 agonists inhibited sexual behaviour and significantly ($P < 0.001$ for the three agonists) reduced the LQ, compared to pre-injection values noted in the same animals. In the non-receptive animals,which should reveal any stimulatory effects, none of the agonists significantly affected behaviour. The two selective $5HT_{1A}$ and $5HT_7$ antagonists had no effect when given alone in the receptive animals, but in the non-receptive group both exerted a small but significant ($P < 0.05$) stimulatory effect (Table 2). Both antagonists were also successful in preventing the inhibitory effects of 5-HTP, 8-0H DPAT and 5-CT (Table 1).

Experiment 2: The effect of OB priming doses and and repeated OB priming on the behavioural response to 8-0H DPAT and 5-CT

Groups of rats were given either 10 µg or 25 µg OB followed by 0.5 mg progesterone. The two agonists, 8-0H DPAT and 5-CT, were tested 3 times at

Table 1 Inhibitory effect of 5-HT agonists on lordosis in the absence and presence of the selective $5HT^7$ (SB 269970-A) and $5HT^{1A}$ (WAY 100135) antagonists in non-receptive and receptive female rats.

Compound	Non-Receptive		Receptive	
	Lordosis Quotient% +/–SEM			
	Pre-injection	Post-Injection	Pre-injection	Post-injection
5-HTP				
+ saline	12.3 +/- 2.8	11.7+/-2.1(12)	55.7+/-1.24	26.5+/-4.4(11)***
+ SB269970-A	19.7+/- 2.8	30.1+/-3.5(12)*	53.2+/- 1.1	61.1+/-2.2(11)
+ WAY 100135	21.6+/- 2.6	18.2+/-3.2(13)	55.9+/- 1.5	51.1+/-2.4(12)
8-OHDPAT				
+ saline	24.2+/- 3.5	16.9+/- 2.8(14)	59.7+/- 1.4	40.9+/-3.2(14)***
+ SB269970-A	11.1+/-1.3	16.0+/-2.3(13)	52.6+/- 1.1	46.3+/- 2.9(11)
+ WAY 100135	20.9+/- 3.0	29.5+/-4.1(21)	52.5+/- 0.9	55.8+/- 2.2(12)
5-CT				
+ saline	11.1+/- 2.3	15,2+/- 1.9(13)	58.6+/- 1.8	40.4+/-2.6(12)***
+ SB269970-A	18.0+/- 2.2	22.7+/- 2.6(13)	52.7+/- 1.2	58.2+/- 2.1(12)
+ WAY 100135	18.7+/- 2.1	20.4+/- 2.7(13)	52.7+/- 1.3	58.1+/- 2.8(11)

Legend

Rats were primed with 10 ug OB followed by 0.5 mg progesterone sc. Tests for sexual receptivity were carried out before ip administration of SB 269970-A (1mg/kg) or WAY 100135 (5 mg/kg). 20 minutes after SB269970-A or 60 minutes after WAY 100135. Groups were treated I.P with either saline (1 'ml/kg), 5HTP (10 mg/kg), 8OHDPAT (0.5 mg/kg), or 5CT (1 mg/kg).Tests were then repeated 15 minutes after administration of the agonists Before assessing the results the rats were subdivided into non-receptive(LQ < 50%) and receptive (LQ > 50%) according to their LQ observed in the pre-injection test. Figures in brackets indicate the number of rats in the group Comparison of pre-and post-injection results were assessed by the Student paired "t" test: *P < 0.05; ***P < 0.0001

14 day intervals, the animals being freshly steroid-primed for each test and the same group always receiving the same agonist.

The concentration of the OB priming dose significantly influenced the response of the rats towards the inhibitory effect of 8-0H DPAT, with the higher dose of 25 µg OB attenuating the inhibitory effect of 8-0H DPAT compared to that observed after 10 µg OB(1-way ANOVA with repeated measures F(1, 25) = 9.625, p = 0.005; Table 3). This difference was maintained at a similar level over the three fortnightly tests, thus while the concentration of OB had a significant effect on response to 8-0H DPAT the effect of repeating the OB treatment was not significant (F(1, 25) = 0.07, p = 0.79, NS; Table 3). The

Table 2 The effect of the selective $5HT^7$ (SB269970-A) and $5HT^{1A}$ (WAY 100135) antagonists on lordosis in non-receptive and receptive female rats.

Compound	Lordosis Quotient% +/–SEM			
	Non-Receptive		Receptive	
	Pre-injection	Post-Injection	Pre-injection	Post-injection
Saline alone	16.3+/- 1.5	18.3+/- 1.9(13)	61.0+/- 1.6.	58.1+/- 0.3(15)
SB alone	17.2+/- 0.9	22.1+/-2.0(14)*	60.9+/- 1.5	65.1+/- 1.7(13)
Saline alone	17.5+/- 1.0	17.6+/- 1.8(12)	56.6+/- 1.5	55.2+/- 1.9(12)
WAY alone	17.5+/- 1.0	24.9+/-1.8(11)*	58.7+/- 1.5	59.6+/- 2.5(12)

Legend

Rats were primed with 10 ug OB followed by 0.5 mg progesterone S.C. Tests for sexual receptivity were carried out before i.p. administration of SB 269970-A(SB; 1 mg/kg) or WAY 100135 (WAY; 5 mg/kg) and then tested 15 minutes after SB or 60 minutes after WAY Before assessing the results, the rats were subdivided into non-receptive (LQ < 50%) and receptive (LQ > 50%)according to their LQ observed in the pre-injection test. Comparison of pre- and post-injection results were assessed by the Student paired "t" test *P < 0.05

Table 3 The effect of oestradiol benzoate priming dose and repeated priming on the effect of 8-OH DPAT and 5-CT treatment.on lordotic activity expressed as a percentage of the pre-treatment response

Compound	Priming dose of OB	No. in Group	Day 1	Day 14	Day 28
8-OHDPAT	10 ug	13	69.6 +/– 4.3	69.5 +/– 4.1	68.2+/– 3.8
	25 ug	14	78.9 +/– 2.8	78.8 +/– 2.7	79.3 +/– 2.0
5-CT	10 ug	13	73.8 +/– 4.2	87.1 +/– 3.2	86.9 +/– 4.7
	25 ug	14	81.6 +/– 8.3	84.5 +/– 4.3	85.4 +/– 2.8

Legend

Rats were primed with 10 ug or 25 ug followed by 0.5 mg progesterone (S.C) before each test which was carried out 3 times at fortnightly intervals. .8OHDPAT (0.5 mg/kg I.P) or 5CT (1 mg/kg I > P) were injected 15 minutes before each test. Results shown are the post-injection results expressed as a percentage of the pre-injection results.

1-way ANOVA with Repeated Measures was used to assess the significance of difference between the effects of the OB priming doses (P0.005) over the 3 test periods and the repetition of the priming (NS) for the 8 OH DPAT groups. The effect of the priming doses and their repetition were NS for the 5CT treated groups.

experiment was repeated employing 5-CT as the agonist. This compound inhibited the LQ in receptive rats treated with either 10 µg or 25 µg OB plus 0.5mg progesterone. The concentration of the priming dose did not significantly affect the response of the rats to 5-CT ($F(1, 25) = 0.112$, $p = 0.741$, NS), nor did the response change over the three fortnightly primings and tests ($F(1, 25) = 1.46$, $p = 0.27$, NS; Table 3).

Interestingly, the OB priming dose affected the response to the selective $5HT_{1A}$ antagonist, WAY100135. Two groups of rats were injected with either

$10\,\mu g$ OB or $25\,\mu g$ OB and 0.5 mg progesterone and given a pre- and post-WAY 100135 injection test only once. The stimulatory effect of WAY100135 was significantly greater after priming with $25\,\mu g$ OB than $10\,\mu g$ OB ($P < 0.05$). There was no significant effect of the priming doses on the effect of the $5HT_7$ antagonist, SB269970-A.

DISCUSSION

The $5HT_7$ receptor is the most recently discovered subtype. It acts via the G-protein $G\alpha s$ to stimulate adenyl cyclase (AC) and thence cAMP (Barnes and Sharp 1999). It is involved in a variety of functions listed in the Introduction; on some exerting a similar effect to the activation of the $5HT_{1A}$ receptor while on others having the opposite effect (see Introduction). The $5HT_{1A}$ receptor couples negatively with G proteins, $G\alpha_1$ and the family of $G\alpha_0$ ($G\alpha_0$, $G\alpha i_1$, $G\alpha i_3$ and $G\alpha i_2$) (Mannoury la Cour et al; 2006) to inhibit AC and thence cAMP production (Fargin et al., 1991). There are, however, circumstances and sites, when $5HT_{1A}$ activation can participate in stimulation of AC (in the guinea-pig hippocampus) (Hoyer et al., 1994; Thomas et al.,1999). $5HT_{1A}$ receptor activation also stimulates phospholipase C via $G\alpha i_3$ (Fargin et al., 1991) and finally it can induce hyperpolarization by G-protein-induced opening of K+ channels, this being independent of cAMP (Barnes and Sharp 1999).

In spite of the differences in their intracellular signalling pathways, $5HT_{1A}$ and $5HT_7$ receptors are considered to be pharmacologically similar and as mentioned above they do affect a number of functions in a similar manner. They also have mutual ligands, examples being 8-0H DPAT which predominantly binds to $5HT_{1A}$ receptors and has a lesser affinity to the $5HT_7$ subtype and 5-CT which binds with a high affinity to both receptors and is currently the most potent agonist for the $5HT_7$ receptor (Thomas et al., 1999). Thus selective $5HT_{1A}$ and $5HT_7$ agonists are not available, but in contrast, selective $5HT_{1A}$ and $5HT_7$ antagonists exist e.g. WAY 100135 ($5HT_{1A}$) (Fletcher et al., 1993) and SB269970-A ($5HT_7$) (Hagan et al., 2000; Thomas et al., 2000)

In a previous report we have shown that activation of both $5HT_{1A}$ and $5HT_7$ receptors mediate the inhibitory effect of 5-HT on LH release (Siddiqui et al., 2000; 2004). In present study we now compare the effects of stimulation of these two receptor subtypes on female sexual behaviour. It is well established that 8-0H DPAT exerts an inhibitory effect on lordotic activity acting on post-synaptic receptors (Uphouse 2000). As far as we know, the effect of 5-CT on lordosis has not been investigated. In this report we have shown that the two 5-HT agonists (8-OH DPAT and 5-CT) with an affinity for both $5H\,T_{1A}$ and $5HT_7$ receptors as well as 5-HTP with an affinity for all the 5-HT receptors significantly reduced lordotic activity in receptive (LQ > 50%) animals and had no significant effect on the non-receptive subgroup (LQ < 50%). The inhibitory effects of all three agonists in receptive animals were prevented by both the $5HT_{1A}$ antagonist, WAY 100135, and the $5HT_7$ antagonist, SB 269970-A. This indicates that both receptors are involved in regulating female sexual behaviour. In the non-receptive animals treated with 5-HTP, SB269970-A induced a rise in lordotic activity suggesting that the 5-HT$_7$ antagonist revealed a stimulatory effect of 5-HTP.

SB269970-A is a selective 5HT$_7$ antagonist (Thomas et al., 2000) and when administered alone, systemically, to non-receptive rats significantly increased lordotic activity. This suggests that endogenous 5HT$_7$ activity might exert a tonic inhibitory control on female sexual behaviour. Interestingly, SB269970-A given alone does not affect LH release (Siddiqui et al., 2004) so the putative endogenous inhibitory action of 5HT$_7$ activity appears to be selective for female sexual behaviour, at least, compared to gonadotrophin release. WAY 100135 is a selective 5HT$_{1A}$ antagonist but it can also exhibit a partial agonist effect on 5HT$_{1A}$ autoreceptors (Assie and Koek, 1996; Fornal et al., 1996) which might affect (i.e., probably enhance) its antagonistic action. Systemic administration of WAY 100135 alone, like SB269970A, stimulated lordotic activity in non-receptive animals and this indicates that endogenous 5HT$_{1A}$ activity may also exert a tonic inhibitory effect on sexual behaviour. This effect has also been shown after central administration of WAY 100135 (Uphouse et al., 1996). The selective 5HT$_{1A}$ antagonist, WAY 100635 also stimulated lordotic activity after systemic administration (Kishitake and Yamanouchi, 2004).

It is assumed that after 5-HTP is administered peripherally, it passes the blood-brain barrier to be converted within the CNS to 5-HT. In receptive rats an injection of 5-HTP inhibited lordotic activity and this effect was prevented by both WAY100135 and SB269970-A. This inhibitory effect of 5-HTP has been shown before in receptive animals (Hunter et al., 1985) and in that same report 5-HTP had a stimulatory effect on non-receptive rats, probably acting via 5HT$_2$ receptors (Hunter et al., 1985). It is not clear why this latter effect was not seen in the current experiments, except to note that the animals used in these experiments are relatively insensitive to steroid priming (see Methods section), so perhaps they are also less sensitive to other stimulatory influences. It can also be noted that prior administration of SB269970-A revealed the stimulatory effect of 5-HTP.

A number of reports have shown that increasing the OB priming dose attenuates or desensitizes the response of animals to the inhibitory effect of 8-0H DPAT on female sexual behaviour (Jackson and Uphouse, 1996;!998; Trevino et al.,1999). Binding studies indicat that this is not due to any changes in 5HT$_{1A}$ receptor affinity or density (Jackson and Etgen, 2001). It may, however, be due to an oestrogen-induced reduction in the coupling of the 5HT$_{1A}$ receptor to Gi/o-proteins as shown can occur in the cortex, hippocampus and amygdala (Mize and Alper, 2000) .The oestrogen effect may be due to an alteration downstream to the receptor as oestrogen reduces the hypothalamic concentration of certain Gαi/o proteins including Gα_Z Gαi$_1$and Gαi$_3$ which couple with the 5HT$_{1A}$ receptor (Raap et al., 2000).This reduction correlates with a desensitization of the effect of 8OH DPAT, on hormone release, and it is suggested by the authors may be the cause of the reduced effect on sexual behaviour.as well (Raap et al., 2000). In addition, OB in a dose-dependent manner upregulates the RGS ZI protein (regulator of G protein signalling-ZI). This is a $G\alpha_2$-selective RGS protein which accelerates $G\alpha_2$ GTP hydrolysis and regulates the duration of interaction between $G\alpha_2$ proteins and effector systems (Carrasco et al., 2004). The $5HT_{1A}$ receptor reduces AC activity via a number of Gi/o proteins including $G\alpha_2$ (Mannour la Cour et al., 2006) and there is some evidence that the inhibitory effect of 8-0H DPAT on lordosis, is associated with a reduction in AC activity and thence cAMP production (Uphouse 2000). If the action of $G\alpha_2$ protein on effector systems is altered by OB, this may be manifested as a reduction in the inhibitory effect of $5HT_{1A}$ activation on AC activity and thence lordosis. (Carrasco et al., 2004). Our experiments employing 10 and 25 µg OB priming doses support this hypothesis (Jackson and Uphouse, 1996;1998;Trevino et al 1999), as the action of 8-0H DPAT was significantly less after 25 µg OB compared to 10 µg OB. We have also shown that the stimulatory effect of WAY 100135, the $5HT_{1A}$ antagonist, is significantly more effective after 25 µg OB compared to 10µg OB. Thus it seems that while the inhibitory effect of $5HT_{1A}$ activity is attenuated by OB, the stimulatory effect due to blocking $5HT_{1A}$ activity is enhanced by OB. In contrast to their effect on $5HT_{1A}$, OB priming doses had no effect on the action of the predominantly $5HT_7$ agonist (5-CT) or its selective antagonist, SB269970-A. This is presumably because the intra-cellular signalling pathways involved in regulating lordotic activity are different for $5HT_{1A}$ and $5HT_7$ receptors.

Uphouse et al (1999) have also shown that repeated hormonal priming before repeated tests for female sexual activity can desensitize the response to 8-0H DPAT. The interval between hormone treatment has to be at least 3 days and can last up to 7 days; longer periods were not tried (Jackson and Uphouse, 1996; Trevino, 1999). In our experiments we subjected the animals to 3 OB plus progesterone treatments at 14 day intervals and found no effect of the repeated priming. Probably this longer period allowed the system to recover from any changes induced by previous treatments.

In summary, we have shown that $5HT_7$ receptor activation mediates an inhibitory effect on female sexual behaviour and this may be a physiological effect as the selective $5HT_7$ antagonist, SB269970-A exerts an effect on the endogenous system and stimulates behaviour. We have also indicated that while there is an interaction between oestrogen and the response to activation of $5HT_{1A}$ receptors by 8-0H DPAT, this relationship does not exist between oestrogen and the $5HT_7$ receptor.

Acknowledgement

This research was supported by Pakistan Science Foundation Grant S-AKU/BIO (281).

References

Ahlenius, S.N., Fernandez-Gausti, A., Hjorth, S., and Larsson, K. (1986). Suppression of lordosis behavior by the putative 5-HT receptor agonist 8-OH DPAT in the rat. Eur. J. Pharmacol. 124:361-363

Aiello-Zaldivar M, Luine V, Frankfurt M. 5,7-DHT facilitated lordosis: effects of 5-HT agonists. NeuroReport 1992; 3:542–4.

Assie MB, Koek W. Effects of 5-HT1A receptor antagonists on hippocampal 5-hydroxytryptamine levels: (S)-WAY100135, but not WAY 100635, has partial agonist properties. Eur J Pharmacol 1996; 23(304):15–21.

Barnes NM, Sharp T. A review of central 5-HT receptors and their function. Neuropharmacology 1999; 38:1083–152.

Bonaventure P, Nepomuceno D, Kwok A, Chai W, Langlois X, Hen R, et al. Reconsideration of 5-hydroxytryptamine (5-HT)(7) receptor distribution 390 A. Siddiqui et al. / Pharmacology, Biochemistry and Behavior 87 (2007) 386–392 using [(3)H]5-carboxamidotryptamine and [(3)H]8-hydroxy-2-(di-n-propylamino) tetraline: analysis in brain of 5-HT(1A) knockout and 5-HT(1A/1B) double-knockout mice. J Pharmacol Exp Ther 2002; 302:240–8.

Carrasco GA, Barker SA, Zhang Y, Damjanoska KJ, Sullivan NR, Garcia F, et al. Estrogen treatment increases the levels of regulator of G protein signaling-Z1 in the hypothalamic paraventricular nucleus: possible role in desensitization of 5-hydroxytryptamine 1A receptors. Neuroscience 2004; 127:261–7.

Fargin A, Yamamoto K, Cotecchia S, Goldsmith PK, Spiegel AM, Lapetina EG, et al. Dual coupling of the cloned 5-HT1A receptor to both adenylyl cyclase and phospholipase C is mediated via the same Gi protein. Cell Signal 1991; 3:547–57.

Fletcher A, Bill DJ, Bill SJ, Cliffe IA, Dover GM, Forster EA, et al.WAY100135: a novel, selective antagonist at presynaptic and postsynaptic 5-HT1A receptors. Eur J Pharmacol 1993; 237:283–91.

Fornal CA, Metzler CW, Gallegos RA, Veasey SC, McCreary AC, Jacobs BL. WAY-100635, a potent and selective 5-hydroxytryptamine1A antagonist, increases serotonergic neuronal activity in behaving cats: comparison with (S)-WAY-100135. J Pharmacol Exp Ther 1996; 278:752–62.

Gorzalka BB, Mendelson SD, Watson NV. Serotonin receptor subtypes and sexual behavior. Ann N Y Acad Sci 1990; 600:435–44.

Hagan JJ, Price GW, Jeffrey P, Deeks NJ, Stean T, Piper D, et al. Characterization of SB-269970-A, a selective 5-HT(7) receptor antagonist. Br J Pharmacol 2000; 30:539–48.

Harvey MT, Smith RL, May ME, Caruso M, Roberts C, Patterson TG, et al. Possible role for the 5-HT1A receptor in the behavioral effects of REM sleep deprivation on free-operant avoidance responding in rat. Psychopharmacology (Berl) 2004; 176:123–8.

Hedlund PB, Huitron-Resendiz S, Henriksen SJ, Sutcliffe JG. 5-HT7 receptor inhibition and inactivation induce antidepressant-like behavior and sleep pattern. Biol Psychiatry 2005; 58:831–7.

Hery M, Becquet D, Francois-Bellan AM, Deprez P, Fache MP, Hery F. Stimulatory effects of 5HT1A receptor agonists on luteinizing hormone-releasing hormone release from cultured fetal rat hypothalamic cells: interactions with progesterone. Neuroendocrinology 1995; 61:11–8.

Hoyer D, Clarke DE, Fozard JR, Hartig PR, Martin GR, Mylecharane EJ, et al. International Union of Pharmacology classification of receptors for 5-hydroxytryptamine (Serotonin). Pharmacol Rev 1994; 46:157–203.

Hunter AJ, Hole DR, Wilson CA. Studies into the dual effects of serotonergic pharmacological agents on female sexual behaviour in the rat: preliminary evidence that endogenous 5HT is stimulatory. Pharmacol Biochem Behav 1985; 22:5–13.

Jackson A, Uphouse L. Prior treatment with estrogen attenuates the effects of the 5-HT1A agonist,8-OH DPAT, on lordosis behavior. Horm Behav 1996; 30: 145–52.

Jackson A, Uphouse L. Dose-dependent effects of estradiol benzoate on 5-HT1A receptor agonist action. Brain Res 1998; 796:299–302.

Jackson A, Etgen AM. Estrogen modulates 5-HT(1A) agonist inhibition of lordosis behavior but not binding of [(3)H]-8-OH DPAT. Pharmacol Biochem Behav 2001; 68:221–7.

Kishitake M, Yamanouchi K. Effects of highly or relatively selective 5-HT1A receptor agonists on lordosis in female rats. Zool Sci 2003; 20:1133–8.

Kishitake M, Yamanouchi K. Facilitatory effects of WAY-100635, a 5-HT1A receptor antagonist, on lordosis n female rats.Neurosci Lett 2004; 371: 147–51.

Lovenberg, TW, Baron, BM; de Lecca, L et al (1993). A novel adenylyl cyclase-activating serotonin receptor (5-HT$_7$) implicated in the regulation of mammalian circadian rhythms. Neuron 11:449-58.

Lucki I, Singh A, Kreiss DS. Antidepressant-like behavioral effects of serotonin receptor agonists. Neurosci Biobehav Rev 1994; 18:85–95.

Mannoury la Cour C, El Mestikawy S, Hanoun N, Hamon M, Lanfumey L. Regional differences in the coupling of 5-hydroxytryptamine-1A receptors to G proteins in the rat brain. Mol Pharmacol 2006; 70:1013–21.

Maswood N, Caldarola-Pastuszka M, Uphouse L. 5-HT3 receptors in the ventromedial nucleus of the hypothalamus and female sexual behavior. Brain Res 1997; 769:13–20.

McEwen BS, Parsons B. Gonadal steroid action on the brain: neurochemistry and neuropharmacology. Ann Rev Pharmacol Toxicol 1982; 22:555–98.

McCarthy and Becker, (2002). Neuroendocrinology of sexual behavior in the female, in: JB Becker, S.M. Breed love, D, Crews and M.McCarthy (eds). Behavioral Endocrinology, PPA Bradford Book, M IT, Boston.

Mendelson, S.D. (1992). A review and re-evaluation of the role of serotonin in the modulation of lordosis behavior in the female rat. Neuroscience Biobehav.Rev. 16:309-350.

Pfaff, D.W. and D.Modianos. Neural mechanisms of female behavior. In : N.Adler, D.W. Pfaff, R.W.Goy (eds.). Handbook of Behavioral Neurobiology, Plenum, New York, 1985, pp. 423 – 493

Rocha-Gonzalez HI, Meneses A, Carlton SM, Granados-Soto V. Pronociceptive role of peripheral and spinal 5-HT7 receptors in the formalin test. Pain 2005; 117:182–92.

Siddiqui A, Kotecha K, Salicioni AM, Kalia V, Murray JF, Wilson CA.

Serotonin inhibits luteinizing hormone release via 5-HT$_{1A}$ receptors in the zona incerta of ovariectomised, anaesthetised rats primed with steroids. Neuroendocrinology 2000; 72:272–83.

Siddiqui A, Abu-Amara M, Aldairy C, Hagan JJ, Wilson CA. 5-HT$_7$ receptor subtype as a mediator of the serotonergic regulation of luteinizing hormone release in the zona incerta. Eur J Pharmacol 2004; 491:77–84.

Siddiqui A, A Niazi, Shaharyar. S. Facilitation of lordosis behaviour is differentially mediated by 5-HT2 receptor agents in diazepam-tolerant rats. Pakistan Journal of Zoology, 2006, 381(1): 46-57

Sprouse J, Li X, Stock J, McNeish J, Reynolds L. Circadian rhythm phenotype of 5-HT7 receptor knockout mice: 5-HT and 8-OH DPAT-induced phase advances of SCN neuronal firing. J Biol Rhythms 2005; 20:122–31.

Takeda H, Tsuji M, Ikoshi H, Yamada T, Masuya J, Limori M, et al. Effects of a 5-HT7 receptor antagonist DR4004 on the exploratory behavior in a novel environment and on brain monoamine dynamics in mice. Eur J Pharmacol 2005; 518:30–9.

Thomas DR, Middlemiss DN, Taylor SG, Nelson P, Brown AM. 5-CT stimulation of adenylyl cyclase activity in guinea-pig hippocampus: evidence for involvement of 5-HT7 and 5-HT1A receptors. Br J Pharmacol 1999; 128:158–64.

Thomas DR, Atkinson PJ, Ho M, Bromidge SM, Lovell PJ, Villani AJ, et al. Price GW. [(3)H]-SB-269970-A selective antagonist radioligand for 5-HT (7) receptors. Br J Pharmacol 2000; 130:409–17.

Thomas DR, Melotto S, Massagrande M, Gribble AD, Jeffrey P, Stevens AJ, et al. SB-656104-A, a novel selective 5-HT7 receptor antagonist, modulates REM sleep in rats. Br J Pharmacol 2003; 139:705–14.

Trevino A, Wolf A, Jackson A, Price T, Uphouse L. Reduced efficacy of 8-OHDPAT's inhibition of lordosis behavior by prior estrogen treatment. Horm Behav 1999; 35:215–23.

Uphouse L. Female gonadal hormones, serotonin, and sexual receptivity. Brain Res Rev 2000; 33:242–57.

Uphouse L, Montanez S, Richards-Hill R, Caldarola-Pastuszka M, Droge M. Effects of the 5-HT1A agonist, 8-OH DPAT, on sexual behaviors of the proestrous rat. Pharmacol Biochem Behav 1991; 39:635–40.

Uphouse L, Andrade M, Caldarola-Pastuszka M, Jackson A. 5-HT1A receptor antagonists and lordosis behavior. Neuropharmacology 1996; 35:489–95.

Wolf A, Caldarola-Pastuszka M, Uphouse L. Facilitation of female rat lordosis behavior by hypothalamic infusion of 5-HT (2A/2C) receptor agonists. Brain Res 1998; 779:84–95.

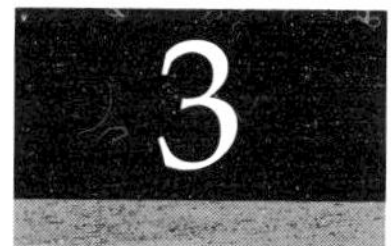

Cerebellar Control of Viscero-motor Activity

O.P. Tandon and Abhinav Dixit

Department of Physiology, University College of Medical Sciences & GTB Hospital,
Dilshad Garden, Delhi-110095

ABSTRACT

The role of cerebellum in the control of somatomotor activities i.e. tone, posture, coordinated movements in form of modulation of lower motor neuron discharges, alpha-gamma linkage interactions with various postural reflexes and neocortex is well documented. In order to effectively control the somatomotor activity, the cerebellum receives inputs from variety of somatic sensory receptors and from higher centres. Afferents from different parts of somites including visceral organs project to the cerebellum on same population of neurons controlling somato and visceromotor activities. There seems to be functional corticonuclear organization in cerebellum from medial to lateral divisions influencing tone, posture equilibrium to coordination of fine manipulatory movements in that order. Different projections of visceral afferents (like somatosensory) in the cerebellum, seem to modify autonomic responses, background visceral reflex activity, visceral smooth muscle tone and vasomotor reflexes including carotid sinus reflexes and autonomic manifestations of sham rage. Recent autonomic and electrophysiological (stimulation, ablation) studies have established the presence of widespread visceral afferent and efferent connections of cerebellum indicating that cerebellum forms a part of supraspinal hierarchy employed in the control of viscero-motor activity. The old concept of parcelation of cerebellum into anterior portion giving viscero-constrictor (sympathotonic) and posterior part, giving viscerodilator (parasympathotonic) responses is no longer valid.

Like somatomotor control of cerebellum on muscle tone, through its facilitatory and inhibitory inputs to descending reticular system, there seems to be efferent pathways for visceromotor modulation through fastigiobulbar tract and its principle relay to spinal cord through paramedian reticular neurons. Though definite muscle spindle afferents and their gamma efferent visceromotor innervation has not been seen in smooth muscle, but it is likely that smooth muscle afferents projecting to cerebellum, through fastigiobulbar tract might influence visceromotor areas of brainstem or lateral horn cells (sympathetic outflow) in the spinal cord, which in turn regulates visceromotor tone. Therefore, it is tempting to assume that on analogy of somatomotor control, cerebellum also regulates by modulating smooth muscle tone, visceral reflexes and vasomotor activity in the bulbar reticular formation regulating visceral activities.

INTRODUCTION

Cerebellum, a part of hindbrain, is known to play well defined roles in motor functions. The shape of cerebellum varies grossly from leaf like e.g. in reptiles to complex shapes as in humans[1]. It is connected by cerebellar peduncles (superior, middle and inferior) to the brainstem. The medial portion is called vermis and the lateral areas, cerebellar hemispheres. Larsell classified the vermis and cerebellar hemispheres using roman numerals. He considered the lobules of hemispheres as extensions of the lobules of the vermis and named them as lobules I to X, with the corresponding lobules of hemispheres being prefixed by H[2]. During ontogeny older portion of cerebellum (archi and paleo) developed simultaneously as limbic structures of cerebral cortex and neocerebellum with neocortex.

Studies on the participation of cerebellum in various functions have been traditionally done by ablation techniques. Later, using of kainic or ibotenic acid gained popularity as a means of chemical ablation. Of late, the method used to study cerebellum and its functions, is electrical stimulation of various cerebellar regions and recording of effects on body systems.

The cerebellar cortex has different types of cells namely Purkinje cells, Golgi cells, granule cells, basket cells and stellate cells. The cerebellar cortex receives afferents from somatic and visceral areas via mossy and climbing fibers as well as diffuse mono-aminergic and cholinergic afferents, sends its output through Purkinje cells to deep cerebellar nuclei, which in turn are connected to neurons in brainstem and cerebrum[1].

CEREBELLUM AND GASTRO-INTESTINAL TRACT

The role of cerebellum in motor activity is now a well established fact[3]. During the last decade, a lot of work has been done in investigating the role of this vital area of brain in non somatic functions i.e. visceral activity, cardiovascular function and cognition[4-6].

Dow in 1939 was among the first to show that stimulation of cutaneous nerves led to cerebellar responses[7]. Later Snider and Stowell demonstrated electrical activity in the anterior lobe of cerebellum following tactile, auditory and visual[8,9]. Widen in 1955, reported potential changes from culmen, simplex and paramedian lobules following stimulation of splanchnic nerves[10]. These potentials were recorded from areas having tactile representation of trunk and extremities, thereby showing that visceral representation occurs in cerebellum.

Newman and Paul (1966), recorded single unit discharges from right side of anterior lobe of cerebellum following distension of gall bladder, mechanical stimulation of abdominal viscera and electrical stimulation of splanchnic nerves[11]. They found that the region of maximum activity was in posterior culmen, lateral to paravermian vein. The authors suggested the possibility of separate viscero-cerebellar pathways from viscera which were independent of somatic sensory pathways. In another study by same persons, splanchnic nerve stimulation activated same areas of cerebellum as electrical stimulation of skin supplied by ninth thoracic segment. This led them to propose that there was convergence of somatic and visceral pathways in cerebellum[12].

Manchanda et al (1972) studied the effect of stimulation of vermis and fastigial nucleus on gastric and duodenal motility[13]. They found that stimulation of the nodule led to increase in tonic and rhythmic contractions of stomach. An increase in cerebellar stimulation led to an increase in gastric motility along with simultaneous decrease in duodenal motility. The response to stimulation of uvula was dependent on the initial state of gastric activity, wherein, at high basal pressure the gastric motility was inhibited and at low pressures, it increased. Martner in 1975 also showed that stimulation of fastigial nucleus affected gastrointestinal motility[14].

Bard in 1947 reported that motion sickness was abolished by removal of certain parts of cerebellum thereby showing that cerebellum participated in visceral functions[15]. Tandon (1971) reported that stimulation of nodule and uvula resulted in increase in gastric acid secretion, substantiating that these areas are involved in motion sickness symptoms[16].

Schmahmann et al (1999) reported an increase in cerebellar blood flow in MRI study on hunger[17]. All these studies thus show that besides being involved in motor activities, cerebellum also plays an important role in gastro-intestinal functioning.

CEREBELLUM AND CARDIORESPIRATORY SYSTEM

Studies done to elucidate the role of cerebellum in cardiorespiratory function revealed that electrical stimulation of fastigial nucleus led to a pressor response, called as, fastigial pressor response. This response was observed in various species like cat, rabbit and monkey[18-20]. This response was abolished following adrenergic blockade or sympathectomy, thereby indicating that it was sympathetically mediated[21-23]. Even the origin of Mayer's waves of blood pressure has been attributed to vermial regions of cerebellum. Both excitation and inhibition of such waves have been reported on cerebellar stimulation[16]. Nisimaru and Kawaguchi found an increase in renal sympathetic nerve activity following stimulation of rostral fastigial nucleus (fastigial pressor area) and caudal fastigial nucleus[24].

A variable pressor or depressor response has been found following electrical stimulation of medial anterior vermis[25-28]. Similar variable response has been reported on stimulation of medial posterior vermis[27,29,30].

Other studies have reported that stimulation of uvula (especially lobule IXb) led to a depressor response in anaesthetized animals and in decerebrate unanaesthetized, a pressor response[31,32].

Recent work has shown that fastigial nucleus, nodulus and uvula modulate respiratory system[31, 33].

All these studies have led to search for the possible pathways for modulation of these activities by cerebellum. Now it is known that cerebellum has connections with various areas of hypothalamus via cerebellar-hypothalamic pathways[34]. The direct connections between cerebellum and hypothalamus were first demonstrated by Dietrichs in 1984[35]. The areas of hypothalamus that project to cerebellum are lateral, posterior and dorsal hypothalamus, mamillary nuclei, dorsomedial and ventromedial nuclei of hypothalamus[34]. These projections are to cerebellar cortex or nuclei alone or to both together. The fibres from cerebellum projecting to hypothalamus arise from various cerebellar nuclei.Through these "to and fro" connections, cerebellum modulates hypothalamic control of visceral and vegetative functions.

CONCLUSION

Cerebellum is not just an area concerned with motor function alone, as believed earlier. Rather it serves as an important area involved in various visceral functions also. The specific location of visceral areas in cerebellum points to a more widespread role of this area and opens new avenues of research.

References

1. Voogd J and Glickstein M. The anatomy of cerebellum. Cerebellum 1998; 21:370-375.

2. Larsell O. The cerebellum, A review and interpretation. Arch Neurol Psychiatr 1937; 31:373-395.

3. Bloedel JR. Cerebellar afferent system: a review. Prog Neurobiol 1973; 2:68.

4. Reis DJ and Golanov. Autonomic and vasomotor regulation. Int Rev Neurobiol 1997; 41:121-149.

5. Scalera G. Effects of corticocerebellar lesions on taste preferences, body weight, food and fluid intake in the rat. J Physiol 1991; 85:214-222.

6. Schmahmann JD and Sherman JC. The cerebellar cognitive affective syndrome. Brain 1998; 121:561-579.

7. Dow RS. Cerebellar action potentials in response to stimuli of various afferent connections. J Neurophysiol 1939; 2:543-555.

8. Snider RS and Stowell A. Evidence of a representation of tactile sensibility in the cerebellum of the cat. Fedn Proc 1942; 1:82.

9. Snider RS and Stowell A. Receieving areas of the tactile, auditory and visual systems in the cerebellum. J Neurophysiol 1944; 7:331-357.

10. Widen L. Cerebellar representation of high threshold afferents in the splanchnic nerve. Acta Physiol Scand 1955; 33 suppl 117:1-69.

11. Newman PP and Paul DH. The representation of some visceral afferents in the anterior lobe of the cerebellum. J Physiol 1966; 182:195-208.

12. Newman PP and Paul DH. The effects of stimulating cutaneous and splanchnic afferents on cerebellar unit discharges. J Physiol 1966; 187:575-582.

13. Manchanda SK, Tandon OP, Aneja IS. Role of the cerebellum in the control of gasto-intestinal motility. J Neural Trans 1972; 33:195-209.

14. Martner J. Cerebellar influences on autonomic mechanisms. An experimental study in the cat with special reference to the fastigial nucleus. Acta Physiol Scand 1975; 425:1-42.

15. Bard P, Woolsey CN, Snider RS, Mountcastle VB, Bromiley RB. Delimitation of central nervous mechanisms involved in motion sickness. Fed Proc 1947; 6:72.

16. Tandon O.P. Exploration of cerebellum in relation to gastrointestinal motility. MD Thesis, All India Institute of Medical Sciences, New Delhi, 1971.

17. Schmahmann JD, Doyon J, McDonald D, Holmes C, Lavoie K, Hurwitz As et al. Three dimensional MRI atlas of the cerebellum in proportional stereotaxic space. Neuroimage 1999; 10:233-260.

18. Achari NK, al-Ubaidy S, Downman CB. Cardiovascular responses elicited by fastigial and hypothalamic stimulation in conscious cats. Brain Res 1973; 60:439-447.

19. Huang TF, Carpenter MB, Wang SC. Fastigial nucleus and orthostatic reflex in cat and monkey. Am J Physiol 1977; 232:H676-681.

20. Bradley DJ, Paton JF, Spyer KM. Cardiovascular responses evoked from the fastigial region of the cerebellum in anaesthetized and decerebrate rabbits. J Physiol 1987; 392:475-491.

21. Achari NK, Downman CB. Autonomic effector responses to stimulation of nucleus fastigius. J Physiol 1970; 210:637-650.

22. Achari NK, al-Ubaidy SS, Downman CB. Spinal sympathoexcitatory pathways activated by stimulating fastigial nucleus, hypothalamus and lower brain stem in cats. Exp Neurol 1978; 62:230-240.

23. Lisander B and Martner J. Interaction between the fastigial pressor response and the baroreceptor reflex. Acta Physiol Scand 1971; 83:505-514.

24. Nisimaru N and Kawaguchi Y. Excitatory effects on renal sympathetic nerve activity induced by stimulation at two distinctive sites in the fastigial nucleus of rabbits. Brain Res 1984; 304:372-376.

25. Stella G and Stevan G. Changes in the heart rate from stimulation of the cerebellar cortex in decerebrate dogs. Arch Int Pharmacdyn Ther 1962; 136:1-11.

26. Rasheed BM, Manchanda SK, Anand BK. Effects of the stimulation of paleocerebellum on certain vegetative functions in the cat. Brain Res 1970; 20:293-308.

27. Nisimaru N, Yamamoto M, Shimoyama I. Inhibitory effects of cerebellar cortical stimulation on sympathetic nerve activity in rabbits. Jpn J Physiol 1984; 34:539-551.

28. Sawyer CH, Hillard J, Ban T. Autonomic and EEG responses to cerebellar stimulation in rabbits. Am J Physiol 1961; 200:405-412.

29. Nisimaru N and Yamamoto M. Depressant action of the posterior lobe of cerebellum upon renal sympathetic nerve activity. Brain Res 1977; 133:371-375.

30. Nisimaru N and Watanabe Y. A depressant area in the lateral nodulus-uvula of the cerebellum for renal sympathetic nerve activity and systemic blood pressure in the rabbit. Neurosci Res 1985; 3:177-181.

31. Bradley DJ, Pascoe JP, Paton JE, Spyer KM. Cardiovascular and respiratory responses evoked from the posterior cerebellar cortex and fastigial nucleus in the cat. J Physiol 1987; 393:107-121.

32. Bradley DJ, Ghelarducci B, Spyer KM. The role of the posterior cerebellar vermis in cardiovascular control. Neurosci Res 1991; 12:45-56.

33. Xu FD and Frazier DT. Modulation of respiratory motor output by cerebellar deep nuclei in the rat. J Appl Physiol 2000; 89:996-1004.

34. Zhu JN, yung WH, Chow BKC, chan YS, Wang JJ. The cerebellar-hypothalamic circuits: potential patheways underlying cerebellar involvement in somatic-visceral integration. Brain Res Rev 2006; 52:93-106.

35. Dietrichs E. Cerebellar autonomic function: direct hypothalamocerebellar pathway. Science 1984; 223:591-593.

4

Intermittent Hypoxia-induced Autonomic Morbidities: An Imbalance in Homeostatic Mechanisms*

Nanduri R. Prabhakar

Center for Systems Biology, Department of Medicine,University of Chicago
Chicago, IL 60637, USA.

ABSTRACT

Chronic Intermittent Hypoxia (CIH) is a life threatening condition that occurs in many different diseases including sleep-disordered breathing manifested as recurrent apnoea. Repetitive, transient cessations of breathing (apnoea) lead to periodic decreases in arterial O_2 saturation and patients with recurrent apnoea develop autonomic morbidities. The purpose of this article is to summarize the cardio-respiratory responses to CIH and the underlying mechanisms. Studies on recurrent apnea patients and rodent models of CIH demonstrated, elevated blood pressures, persistent activation of sympathetic nervous system, elevated plasma catecholamines, altered adrenal medullary responses to hypoxia and ventilatory abnormalities. CIH *up-regulates* chemo-receptor and *down-regulates* baro-receptor reflexes. It is suggested that the imbalance between these two opposing reflex pathways contributes to CIH-induced increases in sympathetic activation, hypertension and respiratory disturbances. Recent studies suggest that reactive oxygen species (ROS)-mediated signaling is a major cellular mechanism associated with CIH-induced autonomic changes. Studies on cell culture models showed that CIH is a potent activator of HIF-1 mediated transcription and involves novel signaling mechanisms. Physiological studies showed absence of cardio-respiratory morbidities in *hif-1a*$^{+/-}$ mice exposed to CIH. ROS were elevated in CIH-exposed wild type mice and this response was absent in *hif-1a*$^{+/-}$ mice. More intriguingly, anti-oxidant not only prevented CIH-induced increases in ROS but also CIH-evoked HIF-1 activation in wild type mice. These results suggest that complex positive

---

*Based on P.B. Sen Oration Award lecture

interactions between ROS and HIF-1 are the up-stream signaling mechanisms that contribute to cardio-respiratory morbidities evoked by CIH.

INTRODUCTION

Adequate availability of oxygen (O_2) is essential for the survival of mammalian cells. Hypoxia, i.e., the decreased availability of O_2, occurs under many different circumstances. Continuous hypoxia (CH) is experienced at high altitudes. Physiological systems adapt during long sojourns at high altitudes. Biochemical and molecular mechanisms underpinning the adaptations to CH are extensively investigated (**4, 32**). People living at sea level experience chronic intermittent hypoxia (CIH) more often than CH. Thus, 50% of premature infants (**27**), 5% of middle aged men and 2% of women after menopause (**22, 33**) experience CIH as a consequence of breathing disorders such as recurrent apneas. Transient repetitive apneas (cessation of breathing) result in periodic hypoxemia (decreases in arterial blood pO_2). Each episode of apnea lasts no more than tenth of a of seconds and the frequency of apneas may exceed 60 episodes per hour with blood hemoglobin saturation of O_2 reduced to as low as 50% in severely affected patients. Unlike, CH, humans experiencing CIH exhibit morbidity of the autonomic nervous system and are prone to develop hypertension, myocardial infarctions and stroke (**22, 33**).Recurrent apneas although results in intermittent hypercapnia (elevations in arterial blood CO_2), exposing experimental animals to CIH alone is sufficient to result in physiological changes similar to those described in recurrent apnea patients (11). Thus, CIH rather than intermittent hypercapnia is the major stimulus for physiological responses to recurrent apneas. The purpose of this article is to summarize the information on physiological responses to CIH and review the recent studies addressing the underlying mechanisms.

AUTONOMIC RESPONSES TO CHRONIC INTERMITTENT HYPOXIA

Cardiovascular and sympathetic responses: Patients with recurrent apneas exhibit elevated blood pressures and sympathetic nerve activity (**5**). Fletcher and his co-workers developed a rodent model of CIH, wherein rats are exposed to alternating cycles of brief episodes of hypoxia (**11**). Rodents exposed to CIH exhibited elevated basal blood pressures and enhanced blood pressure response during acute hypoxic challenge, as well as circulating vasoactive hormones [(i.e., catecholamines, endothelins; (**28**)].

Recurrent apnea patients exhibit elevated sympathetic nerve activity (**5**). Studies on CIH exposed rodents also showed elevated sympathetic nerve activity and enhanced sympathetic excitation during acute hypoxia as well as to hypoxic-hypercapnia. (**34**). Recently Cutler et al (**9**) reported increased muscle sympathetic nerve activity (SNA) in response to voluntary apneas in human subjects and the increased SNA persisted for about 180 minutes. after terminating apneas. Furthermore, addition of CO_2 to the hypoxic stimulus had no significant effect on apnea evoked increases in SNA supporting the idea that hypoxia rather than hypercapnia is the primary stimulus for evoking sympathetic nerve responses. We recently reported that repetitive hypoxia also evokes long-lasting activation of splanchnic SNA in anesthetized rats (**10**). These studies demonstrate that CIH leads to persistent increase in basal sympathetic nerve activity and augmented sympathetic nerve response to acute hypoxia in humans as well as in experimental animals.

Catecholamine secretion from adrenal medulla has been suggested to play an important role in CIH-induced elevations in the blood pressure (**2**). Recently, Kumar et al (**18**) reported that in CIH exposed rats acute hypoxia markedly facilitates catecholamine secretion from adrenal medulla, whereas adrenal medullae from control rats is insensitive to low O_2. The effects of CIH were selective to the hypoxic stimulus because hypercapnia was ineffective in evoking catecholamine secretion from CIH exposed adrenal medullae. CIH-induced hypoxic sensitivity of the adrenal medulla was associated with concomitant down-regulation of neurogenic catecholamine secretion (**18**). On the other hand, prior exposure to CH was ineffective in facilitating hypoxia-evoked catecholamine release from adrenal medulla. The effects of CIH on adrenal medulla are of considerable functional significance in that CIH by down regulating neurogenic catecholamine secretion prevents depletion of catecholamine stores during persistent sympathetic activation, whereas by inducing hypoxic sensitivity, CIH facilitates catecholamine secretion only during hypoxic episodes (i.e., regulated secretion).

Ventilatory responses: CIH in addition to blood pressure also affects breathing. Thus, rats (**24**), mice (**26**) and cats (**31**) exposed to CIH exhibit increased basal ventilations and augmented ventilatory responses to acute hypoxia. Repetitive hypoxia increases breathing and the respiratory stimulation persists as long as an hour after termination of the hypoxic stimulus. The long lasting activation of breathing is a characteristic feature of repetitive hypoxia, because it is not evoked by continuous hypoxia. The persistent elevation of respiration evoked by repetitive hypoxia has been termed as "long-term facilitation" (LTF) of breathing (**21**). Peng & Prabhakar (**24**) reported that CIH potentiates LTF of breathing evoked by acute repetitive hypoxia. The augmented LTF of breathing may explain the increased baseline ventilation seen in CIH exposed animals.

Studies outlined thus far suggest that CIH leads to elevated basal blood pressures, sympathetic nerve activity and ventilation and augments cardio-respiratory responses to acute hypoxia. Furthermore, CIH also leads to remodeling of adrenal medullary function, which might be of significance in evoking cardiovascular responses to CIH.

INTERMITTENT HYPOXIA LEADS TO IMBALANCE BETWEEN CHEMO-AND BARO-REFLEXES

Facilitation of Chemo-reflex by intermittent hypoxia: Peripheral chemoreceptors, especially the carotid bodies are the primary sensory organs for detecting changes in arterial blood oxygen. Reflexes arising from the carotid body mediate autonomic responses including increases in blood pressure, sympathetic activation and breathing. It has been suggested that carotid bodies constitute the "frontline" defense system for detecting systemic hypoxia associated with apneas **(8)**. Consistent with such a possibility were the findings that ventilatory depression with brief hyperoxic challenge (Dejour's test, a measure of peripheral chemoreceptor sensitivity) was more pronounced in obstructive sleep apnea patients than in control subjects **(17)** and that glomectomized subjects with sleep apneas did not develop hypertension **(29)**. Moreover, chronic bilateral sectioning of sinus nerves prevents sympathetic nerve and blood pressures to CIH in rodents **(11)**.

Recent studies provide direct evidence for altered carotid body function by CIH. Hypoxic sensory response of the carotid body was augmented in rats exposed to CIH, whereas hypercapnic sensory response was unaltered **(23)** Sensitization of the hypoxic sensory response of the carotid body was also reported in cats **(31)** and mice **(26)** exposed to CIH. Acute intermittent hypoxia (AIH; 15s of hypoxia followed by 5min of re-oxygenation, 10 episodes) augmented on carotid body sensory activity with each episode of hypoxia and sensory discharge returned promptly to baseline after terminating AIH in control rats. In striking contrast, in CIH exposed animals, sensory activity progressively increased with each episode of AIH, and more importantly, baseline activity remain elevated for about 60min during the post-AIH period. This long-lasting increase in baseline sensory activity has been termed as sensory long-term facilitation (LTF) **(25)**. The effects of CIH on carotid body develop overtime and can be completely reversed after re-exposure of CIH animals to normoxia **(25)**. The reversible nature of the CIH responses might be of considerable clinical significance in that it might explain why treating obstructive sleep apnea patients with nasal continuous positive pressure (nasal CPAP) which reverses cardio-respiratory adverse effects **(17)**. Furthermore, CIH-evoked changes in the carotid body function were not associated with morphological changes in the chemoreceptor tissue **(25)**. These studies demonstrate that CIH results sensitization of the carotid body response to acute hypoxia and long-lasting activation of baseline activity i.e., sensory LTF.

Inhibition of baro-reflex by intermittent hypoxia: Cardio-respiratory responses to a given stimulus not only depend on facilitatory effects from chemo reflexes but also on the inhibitory influence from baro-reflexes. In obstructive sleep apnea patients baro-reflex control of cardiovagal and sympathetic outflow is impaired, and the decreased baro-reflex sensitivity persists even in the wakeful hours **(3, 6)**. Treatment of obstructive sleep apnea with night-time continuous positive airway pressure improves baroreflex function (3). In conscious rats, Lai et al (**19**) found time-dependent decrease in baro-reflex with increasing days of CIH exposures. We examined baro-receptor activity and sympathetic baro-reflex in rats. Our results showed that CIH attenuates baro-receptor mediated inhibition of sympathetic nerve activity, and this effect was associated with marked reductions in the slope as well as saturation frequency of carotid baro-afferent activity in response to increased carotid sinus pressures. Taken together, these observations suggest that CIH results in decreased baro-reflex sensitivity, which is in part due to attenuation of baro-afferent activity.

Significance of altered chemo-and baro-reflexes by intermittent hypoxia: It is evident from the above outlined studies that CIH *up-regulates* chemo- and *down-regulates* baro-reflexes. It is likely that the resulting imbalance between these two opposing reflex pathways play a major role in CIH-induced persistent sympathetic activation and hypertension. In addition, the up-regulation of the chemo reflex may further leads to instability of the respiratory control system, perpetuating apneas.

CELLULAR MECHANISMS UNDELYING CARDIO-RESPIRATORY RESPONSES TO INTERMITTENT HYPOXIA

Role of Reactive Oxygen Species (ROS): CIH is characterized by periodic re-oxygenations. It was proposed that reactive oxygen species (ROS) are generated during the re-oxygenation phase of CIH and ROS mediated signaling contribute to physiological responses to CIH. Supporting such a possibility are the findings that CIH increases ROS in the carotid body (**25**), adrenal medulla (**18**), and brainstem (**30**). More importantly, treating CIH exposed rats with anti-oxidants (MnTMPyP; manganese (III) tetrakis (1-methyl-4-pyridyl) porphyrin pentachloride or NAC; N-acetyl cysteine) prevents CIH-induced: a) alterations in carotid body function (**24, 25**), b) down-regulation of baro-reflex as well as baro-receptor sensitivity, c) functional changes in adrenal medulla (**18**), d) elevations in plasma catecholamines (index of sympathetic activation), and e) blood pressure (**18**). These observations suggest that ROS-mediated signaling is a major cellular mechanism associated with CIH-induced cardio-respiratory changes. Obstructive sleep apnea patients also exhibit increased generation ROS (**7, 20, 35**), and anti-oxidant treatment prevent some of the vascular abnormalities in these patients (**13**).

CIH induces imbalance between pro-and anti-oxidants: Cellular mechanisms of ROS generation include inhibition of complex I and III of the mitochondrial electron transport chain (**1**) as well as activation of several oxidases (**14**). Biochemical measurements showed marked down-regulation of mitochondrial complex I but not the complex III in carotid bodies (**25**) as well as in cell cultures exposed to CIH (**36**). Furthermore, studies on mice and cell cultures showed marked up-regulation of NADPH oxidase subunits (**39, and**

Yuan & Prabhakar, 2007, Unpublished observations). CIH leads to down-regulation anti-oxidant enzyme activities (e.g., superoxide dismutase-2 activity; Khan and Prabhakar, 2007, Unpublished observations). Thus, CIH appears to up-regulate pro and down-regulate anti-oxidant mechanisms and resulting imbalance adds to increased ROS generation.

TRANSCRIPTIONAL RESPONSES TO CHRONIC INTERMITTENT HYPOXIA

Hypoxia inducible factor (HIF-1): **A**ctivation of specific genes is an important mechanism by which hypoxia triggers long-term adaptive responses (**4**). The transcriptional activator hypoxia-inducible factor 1 (HIF-1) is a global regulator of oxygen homeostasis, which regulates the expression of over 60 target genes including those encoding erythropoietin (EPO) and vascular endothelial growth factor (VEGF) (**32**). HIF-1 is a heterodimeric protein that is composed of a constitutively expressed HIF-1β subunit and an O_2-regulated HIF-1α subunit. HIF-1 activity is induced by up-regulating the HIF-1α subunit via decreased rate of O_2-dependent proline hydroxylation, ubiquitination, and proteasomal degradation. HIF-1 transcriptional activity is also regulated via O_2-dependent asparginine (Asn) hydroxylation that blocks co-activator recruitment (**32**).

Yuan et al (**37, 38**) examined the effects of IH on HIF-1 activation in rat pheochromocytoma-12 (PC12) cells. These investigators found that IH results in accumulation of HIF-1α protein, and HIF-1 mediated transcriptional activity in a stimulus-dependent manner, two necessary pre-requisites for HIF-1 dependent regulation of down-stream genes.

Mechanisms of HIF-1 activation by IH: IH-induced HIF1α-stabilization involves Ca^{2+}-dependent activation of rapamycin sensitive mTOR (mammalian target of rapamycin) signaling (**37**), whereas Ca^{2+} dependent calmodulin kinases (CaMKs) participate in HIF-1 transcriptional activation by IH via phosphorylation of p300/CBP co-activators (**38**). These observations suggest that Ca^{2+} signaling plays an important role in IH-induced HIF-1 activation.

Physiological significance of HIF-1 activation by IH: Complete HIF-1α deficiency results in embryonic lethality at mid-gestation, whereas $hif1a^{+/-}$ heterozygous (HET) mice, which are partially deficient in HIF-1α expression, develop normally and are indistinguishable from wild type (WT) littermates under normoxic conditions (**16**). We recently studied the effects of CIH on male littermate WT and $hif1a^{+/-}$ HET mice (**26**). Both groups of mice were exposed to either 10 days of CIH or to 21% O_2 (controls). Analysis of cardio-respiratory responses in CIH-exposed WT mice revealed augmented hypoxic ventilatory response, LTF of breathing, elevated blood pressures and increased plasma noradrenaline. In striking contrast these responses were either absent or attenuated in HET mice exposed to CIH. In CIH exposed WT mice, carotid body response to hypoxia was augmented, and acute intermittent hypoxia (AIH) induced sensory long-term facilitation (sLTF), and these responses were absent in CIH-exposed HET mice. ROS were elevated in CIH-exposed WT mice, and this response was absent in HET mice. MnTMPyP, a potent scavenger of superoxide, not only prevented CIH-induced increases in ROS but also CIH-evoked up-regulation of HIF-1α in WT mice. These observations, taken together suggest that IH activates HIF-1 mediated transcription which appears to be critical for evoking cardio-respiratory responses and the effects of CIH involve complex positive interactions between HIF-1 and ROS. What are the HIF-1 target genes that are affected by CIH? Clinical studies indicate that recurrent apneas are associated with increased serum levels of EPO (**15**) and VEGF (**12**), two target genes activated by HIF-1. Future studies, however, are needed to identify the HIF-1 regulated downstream genes other than EPO and VEGF that potentially contribute to CIH-evoked autonomic changes.

Acknowledgements

The studies are supported by National Institutes of Health, Heart, Lung and Blood Institute Program Project Grant HL-25830, and RO1 HL-076537.

References

1. Ambrosio G, Zweier JL, Duilio C, Kuppusamy P, Santoro G, Elia PP, Tritto I, Cirillo P, Condorelli M & Chiariello M. Evidence that mitochondrial respiration is a source of potentially toxic oxygen free radicals in intact rabbit hearts subjected to ischemia and reflow. J Biol Chem 268, 18532-18541, 1993.

2. Bao G, Metreveli N, Li R, Taylor A and Fletcher EC. Blood pressure response to chronic episodic hypoxia: role of the sympathetic nervous system. J Appl Physiol 83: 95–101, 1997.

3. Bonsignore MR, Parati G, Insalaco G, Marrone O, Castiglioni P, Romano S, Di Rienzo M, Mancia G & Bonsignore G. Continuous positive airway pressure treatment improves baroreflex control of heart rate during sleep in severe obstructive sleep apnea syndrome. Am J Respir Crit Care Med 166: 279–286, 2002.

4. Bunn HF, Poyton RO. Oxygen sensing and molecular adaptation to hypoxia. Physiol Rev. 76, 839-85, 1996.

5. Carlson JT, Hedner J, Elam M, Ejnell H, Sellgren J & Wallin BG. Augmented resting sympathetic activity in awake patients with obstructive sleep apnea. Chest 103, 1763-1768, 1993.

6. Carlson JT, JA Hedner, J Sellgren, M Elam, and BG Wallin. Depressed baroreflex sensitivity in patients with obstructive sleep apnea. Am J Respir Crit Care Med 154: 1490-1496, 1996.

7. Christou K, Markoulis N, Moulas AN, Pastaka C & Gourgoulianis KI. Reactive oxygen metabolites (ROMs) as an index of oxidative stress in obstructive sleep apnea patients. Sleep Breath. 7, 105-10, 2003.

8. Cistulli PA, and Sullivan CE. Pathophysiology of sleep apnea. In: Sleep and Breathing, Edited by Saunders NA, and Sullivan CE. New York, NY: Dekker, 1994, pp. 405–448.

9. Cutler MJ, Swift NM, Keller DM, Wasmund WL, Burk JR & Smith ML. Periods of intermittent hypoxic apnea can alter chemoreflex control of sympathetic nerve activity in humans. Am J Physiol Heart Circ 287, H2054-2060, 2004.

10. Dick TE, Hsieh YH, Wang N, and Prabhakar N.Acute intermittent hypoxia increases both phrenic and sympathetic nerve activities in the rat. Exp Physiol 92: 87-97, 2007.

11. Fletcher EC. Physiological consequences of intermittent hypoxia: systemic blood pressure. J Appl Physiol. 90, 1600-5, 2001.

12. Gozal D, Lipton AJ, Jones KL. Circulating vascular endothelial growth factor levels in patients with obstructive sleep apnea.Sleep. 25:59-65, 2002.

13. Grebe M, Eisele HJ, Weissmann N, Schaefer C, Tillmanns H, Seeger W, and Schulz R. Antioxidant vitamin C improves endothelial function in obstructive sleep apnea. Am J Respir Crit Care Med 173: 897-901, 2006.

14. Halliwell B & Gutteridge JM. Role of free radicals and catalytic metal ions in human disease: an overview. Methods Enzymol 186, 1-85, 1990.

15. Heinicke K, Prommer N, Cajigal J, Viola T, Behn C, Schmidt W. Long-term exposure to intermittent hypoxia results in increased hemoglobin mass, reduced plasma volume, and elevated erythropoietin plasma levels in man. Eur J Appl Physiol. 88:535-43, 2003.

16. Iyer NV, Kotch LE, Agani F, Leung SW, Laughner E, Wenger RH, Gassmann M, Gearhart JD, Lawler AM, Yu AY & Semenza GL (1998). Cellular and developmental control of O2 homeostasis by hypoxia-inducible factor 1 alpha. Genes Dev 12,149-162.

17. Kara T, Narkiewicz K and Somers VK. Chemoreflexes – physiology and clinical implications. Acta Physiol Scand 177: 377–384, 2003.

18. Kumar GK, Rai V, Sharma SD, Ramakrishnan DP, Peng YJ, Souvannakitti D, and Prabhakar NR. Chronic intermittent hypoxia induces hypoxia-evoked catecholamine efflux in adult rat adrenal medulla via oxidative stress. J Physiol 575: 229-239, 2006.

19. Lai CJ, CCH Yang, YY Hsu, YN Lin, and TBJ Kuo. Enhanced sympathetic outflow and decreased baroreflex sensitivity are associated with intermittent hypoxia-induced systemic hypertension in conscious rats. J Appl Physiol 100: 1974-1982, 2006.

20. Lavie L, Vishnevsky A, and Lavie P. Evidence for lipid peroxidation in obstructive sleep apnea. Sleep 27: 123–128, 2004.

21. Mitchell GS, and Johnson SM. Neuroplasticity in respiratory motor control. J Appl Physiol 94: 358-374, 2003.

22. Nieto FJ, Young TB, Lind BK, Shahar E, Samet JM, Redline S, D'Agostino RB, Newman AB, Lebowitz MD, Pickering TG. Association of sleep-disordered breathing, sleep apnea, and hypertension in a large community-based study. Sleep Heart Health Study. JAMA 283,1829-1836, 2000.

23. Peng YJ, and Prabhakar NR. Effect of two paradigms of chronic intermittent hypoxia on carotid body sensory activity. J Appl Physiol 96: 1236–1242, 2004.

24. Peng YJ, and Prabhakar NR. Reactive oxygen species in the plasticity of respiratory behavior elicited by chronic intermittent hypoxia. J Appl Physiol 94: 2342-2349, 2003.

25. Peng YJ, Overholt JL, Kline D, Kumar GK, and Prabhakar NR. Induction of sensory long-term facilitation in the carotid body by intermittent hypoxia:

implications for recurrent apneas. Proc Natl Acad Sci USA 100: 10073-10078, 2003.

26. Peng YJ, Yuan G, Ramakrishnan D, Sharma SD, Bosch-Marce M, Kumar GK, Semenza GL, and Prabhakar NR. Heterozygous HIF-1alpha deficiency impairs carotid body-mediated systemic responses and reactive oxygen species generation in mice exposed to intermittent hypoxia. J Physiol 577: 705-716, 2006.

27. Poets CF, Samuels MP, Southall DP. Epidemiology and pathophysiology of apnoea of prematurity. Biol Neonate. 65, 211–219, 1994.

28. Prabhakar NR, Dick TE, Nanduri J, Kumar GK. Systemic, cellular and molecular analysis of chemoreflex-mediated sympathoexcitation by chronic intermittent hypoxia. Exp Physiol. 92:39-44, 2007.

29. Prabhakar NR. Oxygen sensing during intermittent hypoxia: cellular and molecular mechanisms.J Appl Physiol. 90:1986-94, 2001.

30. Ramanathan L, Gozal D & Siegel JM. Antioxidant responses to chronic hypoxia in the rat cerebellum and pons. J Neurochem 93, 47-52, 2005.

31. Rey S, Del Rio R, Alcayaga J & Iturriaga R (2004). Chronic intermittent hypoxia enhances cat chemosensory and ventilatory responses to hypoxia. J Physiol 560, 577 - 586.

32. Semenza GL. Perspectives on oxygen sensing. Cell 6, 281-4, 1999.

33. Shahar E, Whitney CW, Redline S, Lee ET, Newman AB, Javier Nieto F, O'Connor GT, Boland LL, Schwartz JE, Samet JM. Sleep-disordered breathing and cardiovascular disease: cross-sectional results of the Sleep Heart Health Study. Am J Respir Crit Care Med. 163(1), 19-25, 2001.

34. Sica AL, Greenberg HE, Ruggiero DA, and Scharf SM. Chronic-intermittent hypoxia: a model of sympathetic activation in the rat. Respir Physiol 121: 173–184, 2000.

35. Suzuki YJ, Jain V, Park AM & Day RM. Oxidative stress and oxidant signaling in obstructive sleep apnea and associated cardiovascular diseases. Free Radic Biol Med. 40, 1683-92, 2006.

36. Yuan G, Adhikary G, McCormick AA, Holcroft JJ, Kumar GK & Prabhakar NR. Role of oxidative stress in intermittent hypoxia-induced immediate early gene activation in rat PC12 cells. J Physiol 557, 773-783, 2004.

37. Yuan G, J Nanduri, Semenza G and Prabhakar NR. Mechanisms of HIF-1 stabilization by intermittent hypoxia: Role of Ca2+-mTOR signaling FASEB J. 20, 2006.

38. Yuan G, Nanduri J, Bhasker CR, Semenza GL, and Prabhakar NR. Ca2+/calmodulin kinase-dependent activation of hypoxia inducible factor 1 transcriptional activity in cells subjected to intermittent hypoxia. J Biol Chem 280: 4321–4328, 2005.

39. Zhan G, Serrano F, Fenik P, Hsu R, Kong L, Pratico D, Klann E, and Veasey SC. NADPH oxidase mediates hypersomnolence and brain oxidative injury in a murine model of sleep apnea. Am J Respir Crit Care Med 172: 921-929, 2005.

5

Melatonin in Depressive Disorders – Role of Agomelatine

V. Srinivasan

Department of Physiology, School of Medical Sciences
University Sains Malaysia
16150, Kubang kerian, Kelantan, MALAYSIA

ABSTRACT

Melatonin is the major hormone secreted not only from the pineal gland but also in many other tissues of the body like eye, gastrointestinal tract, thymus, lymphocytes, skin, ovary, platelets, etc. It participates in many functions of the body as regulator a circadian-rhythms, sleep-wake rhythms, as an antioxidant and free radical scavenger, as an effective-hypnotic agent, anti-cancer substance, as a neuroprotector and also in the regulation of mood and behaviour. Melatonin participates in many of these physiological functions by acting through membrane melatonergic receptors like MT_1 MT_2 and MT_3 receptors. It also acts through nuclear orphan receptors in some of the functions. Of the various functions, the role of melatonin in the regulation of human mood has assumed significance in recent years. Numerous studies have substantiated a deficiency of melatonin secretion in depressives although in some studies either low or high melatonin levels have been documented. In addition to changes in the amplitude of diurnal or nocturnal melatonin secretion, melatonin rhythm is also found altered in depressives.Phase shift of melatonin secretion is recognized as prominent feature in major depressive disorder, or seasonal affective disorder. Although changes in both the amplitude and rhythm of melatonin secretion has been documented in patients with major depressive disorder, bipolar disorder, seasonal affective disorder, the use of melatonin as drug in the treatment of patients with mood disorders has met with little success. In this context the development of a novel melatonergic agonist on MT_1 and MT_2 melatonin receptors with $5\text{-}HT_{2c}$ antagonistic properties (agomelatine) has revolutionized the treatment modalities in depressive disorders. Agomelatine in doses of 25 mg/day has been shown to be effective in treating patients with major depressive disorder, bipolar

> disorder and seasonal affective disorder (SAD) in multicenter collaborative studies undertaken in Euriope. It has earlier onset of action, and as an antidepressant reduced the depressive symptoms score, improved sleep efficiency and continuity. Its antidepressant action has been attributed to its effect on MT_1 and MT_2 melatonergic receptors present in the SCN and its antagonistic properties on $5-HT_{2c}$ receptors in the frontal and limbic cortical regions.Agomelatine is unique since it has both sleep regulating effect and mood elevating effect that is not seen with other antidepressants.

INTRODUCTION

Depressive disorders which comprise of major depressive disorder (MDD), bipolar disorder, and seasonal affective disorder constitute a group of psychiatric disorders in which pathological alterations in mood and psychomotor disturbances dominate the clinical picture. Periodic episodes of depression and mania are said to be triggered by changes in the functioning of the master biological clock located located in the anterior hypothalamus. Number of animal studies and clinical studies have shown clearly that the pineal hormone melatonin acts as "arm of biological clock". Clinical studies undertaken in Depressive patients reveal that the onset, offset, amplitude and the rhythm of melatonin secretion is found altered in patients with major depressive disorder, bipolar affective disorder and seasonal affective disorder (Wetterberg et al 1979;[1] Venkoba rao et al, 1983;[2] Arendt, 1989[3]; Tuunainen et al, 2002[4], Crasson et al, 2004)[5].

Melatonin is involved in number of functions of our body like regulation of sleep and circadian rhythms, regulation of reproductive functions, control of mood and behaviour, as a free radical scavenger and anti-oxidant, immune modulator, oncostatic substance (Pandi-Perumal et al, 2006)[6]. A brief introduction about its biosynthesis, regulation of secretion and melatonin receptors will be helpful in understanding its role in the pathophysiology of depressive disorders.

MELATONIN, ITS BIOSYNTHESIS AND REGULATION OF SECRETION

Melatonin is synthesized mainly in the pineal gland of all mammals but its synthesis has been documented in many other areas of our body like the skin, gastrointestinal system, eyes, lymphocytes, thymus gland where the enzymatic machinery involved in melatonin synthesis has been identified. Melatonin is synthesized from the amino acid tryptophan and is converted into 5-hydroxytryptophan and then into 5-hydroxytryptamine or serotonin. Serotonin is then acetylated to form N acetylserotonin by the enzyme arylakylamine-N-acetyltransferease (AA-NAT). N-acetylserotonin is then converted into melatonin by the enzyme hydroxyl indole–O-methyl transferase (HIOMT). Pineal melatonin rhythm exhibits a circadian rhythm with low levels during

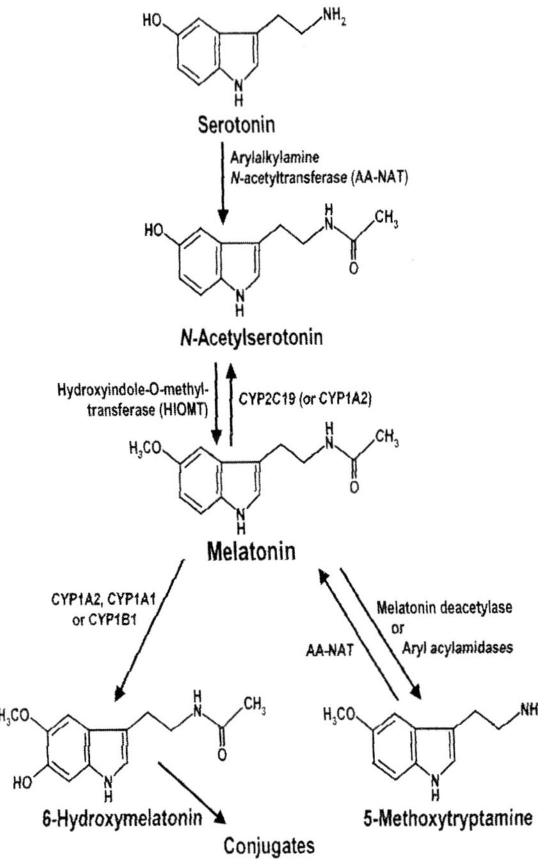

Fig. 1 Melatonin Biosynthesis and Metabolism

daytime and high levels during dark phase of the light-dark cycle. This rhythm is exhibited in all body fluids like plasma, CSF, Urine. The plasma melatonin rhythm has been found remarkably constant and occurs with invariant regularity from day to day and week to week. Melatonin rhythm is synchronized to a 24 day/night cycle by light acting through the retinohypothalamic pathway in animals and human beings. (Moore, 1997)[7]. Special photoreceptive retinal ganglion cells containing melanopsin as a photopigment are involved in this projections (Berson et al, 2002)[8].

Fibers from the SCN pass through the circuitous pathway to reach the intermediolateral horn cells of the spinal cord, which constitute the preganglionic sympathetic neurons for the superior cervical ganglion cells. (Figure 1). The postganglionic sympathetic fibers of the superior cervical ganglion terminate on the pinealocytes and regulate melatonin synthesis by releasing norepinephrine. During the dark phase of the daily photoperiod, the SCN electrical activity being low, the norepinephrine secretion from the sympathetic fibers becomes high thereby stimulating melatonin production from the pineal gland. Norepinephrine by binding with β–adrenergic receptors on the pinealocytes activates adenyl cyclase -cyclic AMP mechanism and promotes melatonin synthesis by activating melatonin–synthesizing enzymes. Once formed melatonin is released into the blood or CSF immediately and its half life is short (20-30 minutes).

Circulating melatonin is metabolized mainly in the liver, where it is first hydroxylated in C6 position by cytochrome P_{450} mono-oxygenases and is conjugated with sulfate and excreted as 6-sulfatoxymelatonin. Melatonin is also metabolized nonenzymatically in all other cells of the body and extracellularly by free radicals to form cyclic 3-hydroxymelatonin (Tan et al, 1998)[9]. In the brain melatonin is metabolized to kynuramine derivatives forming N^1-acetyl-N^2-formyl-5-methoxykynuramine (AFMK). Melatonin since it is both water soluble and lipid soluble diffuses through biological membranes with ease and exerts its actions on almost every cell in the body.

MELATONIN RECEPTORS

Melatonin exerts its physiological actions through membrane bound MT_1 and MT_2 and MT_3 melatonin receptors, nuclear orphan receptors like ROR α 1, RORα 2 and RZRβ. MT_1 and MT_2 are membrane bound receptors and belong to the superfamily of G-protein coupled receptors.

MELATONIN IN MAJOR DEPRESSIVE DISORDER

The interest of melatonin in the pathophysiology of major depressive disorder came ever since Wetterberg and his associates (1979)[1] formulated low melatonin syndrome in Depressive disorders. Number of studies reported low melatonin secretion in depressives(Venkoba rao et al, 1983;[2] Claustrat et al 1984;[10] Nair et al, 1984;[11] Brown et al, 1985[12]; Sack and Lewy 1988[13]; Paparrigopoulos et al, 2001)[14]. In some studies clinical symptoms such as suicidal ideas correlated with decrease in melatonin levels (Venkoba rao et al, 1983)[2]. Dysfunctionality of melatonin secretion in major depressive disorders included increase in melatonin secretion (Rubin et al, 1992;[15] Crasson et al, 2004)[5] The increased melatonin levels reported in these patients could be a compensatory mechanism in response to decreased melatonin receptor density, although direct evidences for such thing is yet to be reported. In addition to rhythm of secretion, melatonin 's phase position is also affected in depression. Phase advancement of melatonin rhythm has been reported in depressives (Beck-Friis et al, 1985[16] Nair et al, 1984;[11] Claustrat et al 1984;[10] Wehr et al, 1985)[17].

ANTIDEPRESSANT TREATMENT ON MELATONIN SECRETION IN MAJOR DEPRESSIVE DISORDER

Treatment of depressive patients with tricyclic antidepressant like imipramine has been shown to increase melatonin levels (Venkoba rao et al, 1983;[2] Thompson et al, 1985[18]; Brown et al, 1985(b)[19] Sack and Lewy, 1986;[20] Golden et al 1988).[21] The clinical evidence showing that antidepressant treatment changes melatonin secretion in patients with major depressive disorder suggests that pineal gland plays a role in the etiology of mood disorders. Experimental studies undertaken in rats involving psychotherapeutic drugs like imipramine, monoamine oxidae inhibitors (MAOI) diazepam, chlorpromazine have all shown that they all increase pineal melatonin content (Srinivasan, 1989)[22].

ROLE OF MELATONIN IN BIPOLAR AFFECTIVE DISORDERS

Bipolar affective disorders are characterized by the occurrence of mania, or hypomania either preceded or followed by depression. Number of studies in bipolar patients have revealed that there is disturbance in their circadian rhythms including sleep-wake cycles and this has been suggested to be due to dysfunctioning of SCN–pineal link. (Srinivasan et al, 2006)[23]. Reduced amplitude of melatonin secretion has been found in bipolar depressed patients during depressive phase (Souetre et al, 1989)[24]. In another study reduced melatonin secretion has been found during depressive, manic and euthymic states of bipolar depressive patients (Kennedy et al, 1996)[25] suggesting thereby that decreased melatonin secretion may be a trait marker in bipolar disorders.

BRIGHT LIGHT AND MELATONIN SUPPRESSION IN BIPOLAR DEPRESSIVES

Lewy et al (1980)[26] first demonstrated that light intensity of 500 lux suppresses plasma melatonin levels in human beings. In a subsequent study undertaken Lewy and his coworkers further showed that exposure to 500 lux bright light caused 50% suppression of plasma melatonin levels in bipolar patients while it did not cause any suppressive effects in normal controls. In a recent study it was observed that exposure to bright light to bipolar I disorder exhibited greater suppression of melatonin (62.7%) as compared to matched controls (40.0%) These findings suggest that excessive light-induced suppression may be a risk factor for the development of bipolar affective disorder (Nurnberger et al, 2000[27].

MELATONIN IN SEASONAL AFFECTIVE DISORDER

Seasonal affective disorder or Winter depression is chareceterized by recurrent episodes of depression during winter months and Euthymia or hypomania in Spring or summer. Patients suffering from this disorder exhibit symptoms like hypersomnia, hyperphagia, carbohydrate craving and weight gain (Rosenthal et al, 1984[28]). Lewy (1987)[29] first reported phase delay of circadian rhythms in patients with seasonal affective disorders and this has been proved subsequently by many other investigators (Sack et al, 1990;[30] Dahl et al, 1993[31]; Avery et al, 1997)[32].

TREATMENT OF DEPRESSIVE DISORDERS: CURRENT CHOICE

Depressive disorders account for the fourth leading cause of global burden of disease and by the year 2020 they are expected to be the second highest cause of morbidity (Lecrubier, 2001)[33]. In the early 1960s MAOIs and tricyclic antidepressants have been the drugs of choice for treating depressive disorders. While MAOIs have not been popular, tricyclics have been preferred. But their use also has been associated with the risk of adverse side effects like cardiotoxicity, anticholinergic side effects, weight gain etc. (Owens, 1994). Subsequently new generations of antidepressants like SNRIs (serotonin –noradrenaline reuptake inhibitors) SSRIs (selective serotonin reuptake inhibitors) have emerged.These drugs offered modest advantage over tricyclics in terms of tolerability. The efficacy of SSRIs in treating severe depression has been shown to vary from 53 to 64% compared to 43% to 70% observed for tricyclics. (Hirscfeld, 1999)[34]. But superior efficacy of an antidepressant rests primarily on an earlier onset of action and improved clinical effect (Loo et al, 2002). Both SNRIs and SSRIs have only limited efficacy in treating severe depression and moreover they have a long latency period (Clerc, 2001)[35]. Since sleep and circadian rhythm dysregulation constitute integral features of affective disorders, a drug that has an effect in improving both sleep and circadian rhythm dysregulation will have greater beneficial effect in treating patients with affective disorders than the conventional antidepressant drugs. The currently prescribed antidepressants in fact have adverse effects on sleep and in fact insomnia is often worsened by antidepressant treatment (Lam, 2006)[36].

AGOMELATINE, THE NOVEL MELATONERGIC ANTIDEPRESSANT

Agomelatine is newly developed melatonergic antidepressant and is both an $MT_1/$ MT_2 melatonin receptor agonist and is also a selective antagonist of 5-hydroxytryptamine $(5\text{-HT})_{2c}$ receptors. It is chemically designated as N-[2-(7-methoxynaphth-1-yl)acetamide. Agomelatine displays a greater affinity (over 100 fold) to MT_1/MT_2 receptors than melatonin. It has no significant affinity for muscarinic, histaminergic, adrenergic, or dopaminergic receptor subtypes (Rouillon, 2006)[37]. In animal studies it was proved that agomelatine is able to resynchronize the disrupted circadian rhythms and this effect is attributed predominantly to its action on MT_1/MT_2 receptor sites in the suprachiasmatic nucleus of the hypothalamus (Turek and Gillette, 2004)[38].

AGOMELATINE EFFECTS IN ANIMAL MODELS OF DEPRESSION

Agomelatine has been found effective in alleviating the symptoms of depression in several animal models of depression like learned helplessness test, forced swimming test, psychosocial stress in tree shrews, in mild stress model (Papp et al, 2003,[39] Pandi-Perumal et al, 2006)[40]. It is suggested that dopaminergic and adrenergic mechanisms in the frontal cortex modulate mood and cognition.

These functions are severely affected in depressive illness. The therapeutic efficacy of agomelatine has been attributed partly due to its action of releasing norepinephrine, and dopamine in the frontal cortex (Millan et al, 2003). The 5-HT_{2c} antagonistic properties of agomelatine are largely responsible for the enhancement of frontal dopaminergic and adrenergic transmission.

AGOMELATINE IN MAJOR DEPRESSIVE DISORDER

Number of clinical studies have been undertaken by using agomelatine in patients with major depressive disorder. In a multicenter, multinational, placebo controlled study involving 711 patients from 102 centers located in Belgium, France and UK it was found that administration of agomelatine in the dose of 25 mg/day for a period of 8 weeks, reduced the depressive symptoms significantly as revealed by the findings of Hamilton depression rating score for depression. Significantly in patients with severe depression scores also agomelatine in doses ranging from 25 to 50 mg/day, reduced depression scores significantly (P < 0.05).) (Loo et al, 2002[41]). In this study it was found that agomelatine exhibited good tolerability, and safety. The frequency of side effects such as headache, abdominal pain, diarrhea observed with agomelatine were lower than that of placebo administration. In a similer study involving 212 outpatients from Canada, South Africa also, it was found that agomelatine was effective (25 mg/day) in reducing depressive scores significantly when administered for the duration of 6 weeks.(Kennedy et al, 2006)[42] Agomelatine also exhibited superior efficacy while treating severely depressed patients in this study also. This supports the inference that agomelatine may have a superior therapeutic potential when compared with other currently prescribed antidepressants. (Pandi-Perumal et al, 2006)[40].

AGOMELATINE IN BIPOLAR DISORDER

Sleep disturbances are the most common symptoms for major depressive disorder and constitute one of the diagniostic criteria for major depressive disorder. Most antidepressants often worsen the sleep problems and hence require concomitant administration of hypnotic drugs as adjunct therapy. Agomelatine within a week after its administration improved subjective sleep onset and sleep quality when compared with venlafaxine (Guilleminault, 2005)[43]. In a recent study conducted on 21 Bipolar I (depressed) patients, administration of 25 mg of agomelatine for more than 6 weeks was found effective in reducing the depressive scores significantly. It also exhibited greater efficacy and safety (Calabrese et al, 2007)[44].

AGOMELATINE IN SEASONAL AFFECTIVE DISORDER

Besides being effective in treating patients with major depressive disorder (MDD), Bipolar Depressed patients, agomelatine also has been found effective in treating patients with Seasonal depression. In a recent study conducted on 37 acutely depressed SAD patients administration of agomelatine (25 mg/day) for a period of 14 weeks, reduced significantly SIGH-SAD, CGI-5, CGI-1 scores from second week onwards (P < 0.001). A significant factor of this study was that throughout the period of study over 14 weeks, agomelatine exhibited good tolerability and from this study it was concluded that agomelatine, the first melatonergic antidepressant is also effective in treating patients with seasonal depression. (Pjrek et al, 2007) [45]

CONCLUSION

Clinical studies undertaken in patients with mood disorders have shown clearly that both the rhythm and amplitude of melatonin secretion in patients with major depressive disorder, bipolar affective disorder and seasonal affective disorder. This suggests that either abnormal melatonin secretion or abnormal functioning of melatonin receptors are involved in the pathophysiology of mood disorders. Psychopharmacological studies undertaken in animals have shown that administration of antidepressants stimulate pineal melatonin production. Similarly clinical studies involving patients with affective disorders also have revealed that antidepressant administration in them is followed by marked changes in either plasma melatonin or urinary 6-sulfatoxy melatonin excretion or both. Since most of the antidepressants that are currently prescribed cause marked sleep disturbances and sleep disturbances constitute one of the major clinical features of depressive illness, the need to improve sleep efficiency has become the major target for antidepressants. Concomitant administration of hypnotic drugs has been in use for alleviating sleep problems in patients with mood disorders. However use of these hypnotic drugs cause hangover effects in the next day morning also. Now the introduction of novel me; atonergic antidepressant agomelatine that has more affinity for MT_1 MT_2 receptors with $5\text{-}HT_{2c}$ antagonistic properties has been found beneficial in treating patients with major depressive disorders, bipolar disorder, and seasonal affective disorder. The drug has been found efficient in reducing depressive scores, and improving sleep problems very well. Fortunately it did not exhibit any of the side effects exerted by other antidepressants and has been found safe. However more number of clinical trials with longer duration of more than 6 months are required to substantiate the claims that the drug is safer for long term use.

References

1. Wetterberg L. Clinical importance of melatonin. Prog Brain Res 1979; 52: 539-547.
2. Venkoba rao A, Parvathi devi S, Srinivasan V. Urinary melatonin in depression. Ind J Psychiat 1983; 25 : 167-172.
3. Arendt J. Melatonin : A new probe in psychiatric investigation ? Br J Psychiatry 1989; 155: 585-590.
4. Tuunainen A, Kripke DF, Elliott JA, Assmus JD, Res KM, Klauber MR, Langer RD. Depression and endogenous melatonin in postmenopausal women. J Affect Disorder 2002; 69: 149-158. S

5. Crasson M, Kjiri DJ, Colin A, Kjiiri K, L' Hermite-Baleriaux M, Ansseu M, Legros JJ Serum melatonin and urinary 6-sulfatoxymelatonin in major depression. Psycho-neuroendocrinology. 2004; 29-1-12.

6. Pandi-Perumal SR, Srinivasan V, GJM Maestroni, Cardinali DP, Poeggeler B, Hardeland R. Melatonin : Nature's most versatile signal ? FEBS J 2006; 273: 2813-2838.

7. Moore RY. Circadian rhythms : basic neurobiology and clinical applications. Ann Rev Med 1997; 48: 253-266.

8. Berson DM, Dunn FA, Takao M. Phototransduction by retinal ganglion cells that set the circadian clock. Science 2002; 295: 1070-1073.

9. Tan DX, Manchester LC, Reiter RJ, Plummer BF, Hardies LJ, Weintraub ST, Vijayalaxmi, Shepherd AM. A novel melatonin metabolite, cyclic 3-hydroxymelatonin : a biomarker of in vivo hydroxyl radical generation. Biochem Biophys Res Commun 1998; 253: 614-620.

10. Claustrat B, Chazot G, Brun J, Jordan D, Sassolas G. A chronobiological study of melatonin and cortisol secretion in depressed subjects; plasma melatonin a biochemical marker in major depression.Biol Psychiatry 1984; 19 :1215-1228.

11. Nair NP, Hariharasubramanian N, Pilapil C. Circadian rhythm of plasma melatonin in endogenous depression. Biol Psychiat 1984; 715- 718.

12. Brown R, Kocis JH, Caroff S, Amsterdam J, Winokur A. Stokes PE, Frazer A. Differences in nocturnal melatonin secretion between melancholic depressed patients and control subjects. Am J Psychiatry 1985 (a). 142 : 811- 816.

13. Sack RL, Lewy AJ. Melatonin and major affective disorders. In Miles A, Philbrich D, Thompson C Eds.Melatonin; Clinical perspectives. New york, Oxford Medical publications. pp 205-227, 1988.

14. Paparrigopoulos T, Psarros C, Bergiannaki J, Varsou E, Dafni U, Stefanis C. Melatonin response to clonidine administration in depression.indication of presynaptic alpha$_2$–adrenoceptor dysfunction. J Affective Disorder 2001; 65: 307-313.

15. Rubin RT, Heist EK, McGeoy SS, Hanada K, Lesser IM. Neuroendocrine aspects of primary of primary endogenous depression. XI. Serum melatonin measures in patients and matched controls. Arch Gen Psychiatry 1992; 49: 558-567.

16. Beck–Friis J, Kjellman BF, Aperia B, Unden F, von Rosen D, Ljunggren JG, Wetterberg L. Serum melatonin in relation to clinical variables in patients with major depressive disorder and a hypothesis of low melatonin syndrome. Acta Psychiatr Scand 1985; 71:319-330.

17. Wehr TA, Sack DA, Duncan WC, Mendelson WB, Rosenthal NE,Gillin JC, Goodwin FK. Sleep and circadian rhythms in affective patients isolated from external time cues. Psychiatry Res 1985; 15: 327- 339.

18. Thompson C, Mezey G, Corn T, Franey C, English J, Arendt J, Checkley SA. The effect of desipramine upon melatonin and cortisol secretion in depressed and normal subjects. Br J Psychiatry 1985; 147: 389-393.

19. Brown RP, Koosis JH, Caroff S, Amsterdam J, Winokur A,Stokes P, Frazer A. Nocturnal serum melatonin in major depressive disorder before and after desmethyl treatment. Psychopharmacol Bull 1985; 21: 579-581.

20. Sack RL, Lewy AJ.Desmethylimipramine treatment increases melatonin production in humans. Biol Psychiatry 1986; 21: 406-410.

21. Golden RN, Markey SP, Risby ED, Rudorfer MV, Cowdry RW, Potter WZ. Antidepressants reduce whole-body norepinephrine turnover while enhancing 6-hydroxymelatonin output.Arch Gen Psychiatry 1988; 45: 150-154..

22. Srinivasan V. Psychoactive drugs, pineal gland and affective disorders. Prog Neuropsychopharmacol Biol Psychiatry 1989; 41: 309- 328.

23. Srinivasan V, Smits MG, Spence W, Lowe AD, Kayumov L, Pandi-Perumal SR, Parry B, Cardinali DP. Melatonin in mood disorders. World J Psychiatry 2006;

24. Souetre E, Salvati E, Belugou JL, Pringuey D, Candito M, Krebs B, Ardisson JL, Darcourt G. Circadian rhythms in depression and recovery.Evidence for blunted amplitude as the main chronobiological abnormality.Psychiatr Res 1989; 28: 263-278.

25. Kennedy SH, Kutcher SP, Ralevski E, Brown GM. Melatonin and cortisol 'switches' during mania, depression and euthymia in a drug free bipolar patients. J Nerv Ment Dis 1989; 177: 300-303.

26. Lewy AJ, Wehr TA, Goodwin FK, Newsome DA, Markey SP. Light suppresses melatonin secretion in humans. Science 1980; 210: 1267-1269.

27. Nurnberger JI Jr, Adkins S, Lahiri DK, Mayeda A, Hu K, Lewy AJ, Miller A, Bowman ES, Miller MJ, Rau L, Smiley C, Davis-singh D. Melatonin suppression by light in euthymic bipolar and unipolar patients. Arch Gen Psychiatry 2000; 57:572-579.

28. Rosenthal NE, Sack DA, Gillin JC, Lewy AJ, Goodwin FK, Davenport Y, Mueller PS, Newsome DA, Wehr TA. Seasonal affective disorder. A description of the syndrome and preliminary findings with light therapy. Arch Gen Psychiatry 1984; 41: 72-80.

29. Lewy AJ, Sack RL, Singer CM, White DM. The phase shift hypothesis for bright light's therapeutic mechanism of action.Theoritical considerations and experimental evidence.Psychopharmacol Bull 1987; 23: 349-353.

30. Sack RL,Lewy AJ, White DM, Singer CM, Fireman MJ, Vandiver R. Morning vs evening light treatment for winter depression.Evidence that the therapeutic effects of light are mediated by circadian phase shifts.Arch Gen Psychiatry 1990; 47: 343-351.

31. Dahl K, Avery DH, Lewy AJ,SavageMV, Brengelmann GL, Larsen LH, Vitiello MV, Prinz PN. Dim light melatonin onset and circadian temperature during a constant routine in hypersomnic winter depression. Acta Psychiatr Scand 1993; 88: 60-66.

32. AveryDH, Dahl K, Savage MV, Brengelmann GL, Larsen LH, Kenny MA, Eder DN, Vitiello MV, Prinz PN. Circadian temperature and cortisol rhythms during a constant routine are phase–delayed in hypersomnic winter depression. Biol Psychiatry 1997; 41: 1109-1123.

33. Lecrubier Y. The burden of depression and anxiety in general medicine. J Clin Psychiatry 2001; 62(Suppl 8): 4-9.

34. Hirschfeld RM. Efficacy of selective serotonin reuptake inhibitors (SSRIs) and newer antidepressants in severe depression: Comparison with tricyclic antidepressants (TCAs). J Clin Psychiatry 1999; 60: 326-335.

35. Clerc G. Antidepressant efficacy and tolerability of milnacipran, a dual serotonin and noradrenaline reuptake inhibitor. A comparison with fluvoxamine. Int Clin Psychopharmacol 2001; 16: 145-151.

36. Lam RW. Sleep disturbances and depression : a challenge for antidepressants. Int Clin Psychopharmacol 2006; (Suppl1) S25-S29.

37. Rouillon F. Efficacy and tolerance profile of agomelatine and practical use in depressed patients. Int Clin Psychopharmacol 2006; 21(suppl1) : S31-S35.

38. Turek FW, Gillette MU. Melatonin, sleep,and circadian rhythms.rationale for development of specific melatonin agonists.Sleep Med 2004; 5: 523-532.

39. Papp M, Gruca P, Boyer PA, Mocaer E. Effect of agomelatine in the chronic mild stress model of depression in the rat.Neuropsychopharmacology 2003; 28: 694-703.

40. Pandi-Perumal SR, Srinivasan V, Cardinali DP, Monti JM. Could agomelatine be the ideal antidepressant ? Expert Rev Neurotherapeutics 2006; 6: 1595-1608.

41. Loo H, Hale A, D'haenen H. Determination of the dose of agomelatine, a melatonergic agonist and selective 5-HT(2C) antagonist, in the treatment of major depressive disorder : a placebo controlled dose range study. Int Clin Psychopharmacol 2002; 17: 239-247.

42. Kennedy SH, Emsley R. Placebo controlled trial of agomelatine in the treatment of major depressive disorder. Eur Neuropsychopharmacol 2006; 16: 93-100.

43. Guilleminault C. Efficacy of agomelatine versus venlafaxine in subjective sleep of patients with major depressive disorder.Eur Neuropsychopharmacol 2005; 15 (suppl3) : S 419 (abstract).

44. Calabrese JR, Guelfi JD, Perdrizet-Chevalier C. Agomelatine adjunctive therapy for acute bipolar depression: preliminary open data. Bipolar Disorders 2007; 9: 628-635.

45. Pjrek E, Winkler D, Konstantinidis A,Willeit M, Praschak-Reider N, Kasper S. Agomelatine in the treatment of seasonal affective disorder. Psychopharmacology (Berlin) 2007; 190:575-579.

6

Nickel Toxicities: Role of Oxidative Stress and Protective Antioxidants (L-Ascorbic Acid and Alpha-tocopherol)

Kusal K. Das*, Amrita Das Gupta and Salim A. Dhundasi

Environmental Health Research Unit, Department of Physiology,
Al Ameen Medical College, Bijapur-586108, Karnataka, India

ABSTRACT

on the generation and role of reactive
article. Nickel is a known hematotoxic,
tic, and nephrotoxic agent. This article
its effect on certain metabolically active
in the author's laboratory. The review
eneration of reactive oxygen species and
abolically active tissues, and the possible
s protective antioxidants.

l pollutants, nickel (Ni), a heavy metal, lly toxic element, even though it is an an and animal. Pure nickel is a hard, ies that make it very desirable for lloys e.g. with Fe, Cu, Cr and Zn. The to widespread environmental pollution d disposal. Nickel is released into by industries such as oil-burning power plants, coal-burning power plants, trash incinerators, rubber, and plastic

---

**Corresponding Author*

industries, nickel-cadmium battery industries, and electroplating industries[1]. Nickel in air remains attached to small particles and it ranges from 1-86 ng/m^3. On the other hand the level of nickel in water is often as low as 10 ppb or less (except in industrial areas). Nickel enters the body when breathing air containing nickel, drinking water or eating food that contains nickel, or when skin comes into contact with nickel. Some food contains high concentration of nickel e.g. tea, coffee, chocolate, soybeans, nuts, potatoes, cabbage, spinach etc. absorbed nickel is transported in blood by binding with albumin or histidine or by a plasma protein, called nickeloplasmin[2]. Contrary to insoluble nickel compounds, the soluble salts of nickel are readily absorbed by the pulmonary and digestive tracts, and less by the skin. Nickel is not a cumulative toxicant and most of the absorbed metal is excreted rapidly. Most ingested nickel leaves quickly in the feces, but a small amount can enter the blood and leave in the urine. In the general population, the average nickel concentrations in serum and urine are 0.2 µg/L and 0.1 to 13.3 µg/L, respectively [3, 4]. The adverse health effects of nickel depend on the route of exposure (inhalation, oral, or dermal) and can be classified according to systemic, immunologic, neurologic, reproductive, developmental, or carcinogenic effects following acute (14 days or less), intermediate (15–364 days), and chronic (365 days or more) exposure periods. Based on studies of nickel workers and laboratory animals, all nickel compounds, except for metallic nickel, have been classified as human carcinogens by the International agency for research on cancer (IARC).

HEAVY METALS AS FREE RADICAL GENERATORS

The mechanisms of heavy metals toxicity through electron transfer most often involve the cross linking of the sulfhydryl groups of proteins. Nickel and other heavy metals can also generate free radicals directly from molecular oxygen in a two step process to produce superoxide anion. In the continued presence of the heavy metal, the superoxide anions formed can then combine with protons in the dismutation reaction generating hydrogen peroxide in the process. Although, nickel (II) by itself does not cause efficient free radical generation from oxygen, H_2O_2, or lipid hydroperoxides, the reactivity of Ni (II) with those oxygen derivatives can be modulated by chelation with certain histidine- and cysteine-containing ligands. The incubation of Ni (II) with cysteine in an aerobic environment generates the hydroxyl radical, which then reacts with cysteine to generate a carbon-centered alkyl radical[5]. Free radicals can also be generated from lipid hydroperoxides by Ni (II) in the presence of several oligopeptides.

NICKEL ON HEALTH

In acute toxicity of nickel, there is report of a rise in blood insulin level, a profound increase in serum prolactin level, alteration of several enzymatic

Nickel Toxicities: Role of Oxidative Stress and Protective Antioxidants (L-Ascorbic Acid and Alpha-tocopherol)

Kusal K. Das*, Amrita Das Gupta and Salim A. Dhundasi
Environmental Health Research Unit, Department of Physiology,
Al Ameen Mcdical College, Bijapur-586108, Karnataka, India

ABSTRACT

Nickel-induced toxicity with an emphasis on the generation and role of reactive oxygen species is briefly reviewed in this article. Nickel is a known hematotoxic, immunotoxic, hepatotoxic, pulmonary toxic, and nephrotoxic agent. This article presents a selective review on nickel and its effect on certain metabolically active peripheral tissues which were evaluated in the author's laboratory. The review particularly addresses the nickel-induced generation of reactive oxygen species and increased lipid peroxidation in various metabolically active tissues, and the possible role of L-ascorbic acid and α-tocopherol as protective antioxidants.

INTRODUCTION

Among these myriads of environmental pollutants, nickel (Ni), a heavy metal, merits a special reference as a potentially toxic element, even though it is an essential trace element for both human and animal. Pure nickel is a hard, silvery white metal having properties that make it very desirable for combining with other metals to from alloys e.g. with Fe, Cu, Cr and Zn. The vast industrial use of the metal has led to widespread environmental pollution during its production, recycling and disposal. Nickel is released into atmosphere during nickel mining and by industries such as oil-burning power plants, coal-burning power plants, trash incinerators, rubber, and plastic

---

**Corresponding Author*

industries, nickel-cadmium battery industries, and electroplating industries[1]. Nickel in air remains attached to small particles and it ranges from 1-86 ng/m^3. On the other hand the level of nickel in water is often as low as 10 ppb or less (except in industrial areas). Nickel enters the body when breathing air containing nickel, drinking water or eating food that contains nickel, or when skin comes into contact with nickel. Some food contains high concentration of nickel e.g. tea, coffee, chocolate, soybeans, nuts, potatoes, cabbage, spinach etc. absorbed nickel is transported in blood by binding with albumin or histidine or by a plasma protein, called nickeloplasmin[2]. Contrary to insoluble nickel compounds, the soluble salts of nickel are readily absorbed by the pulmonary and digestive tracts, and less by the skin. Nickel is not a cumulative toxicant and most of the absorbed metal is excreted rapidly. Most ingested nickel leaves quickly in the feces, but a small amount can enter the blood and leave in the urine. In the general population, the average nickel concentrations in serum and urine are 0.2 µg/L and 0.1 to 13.3 µg/L, respectively [3, 4]. The adverse health effects of nickel depend on the route of exposure (inhalation, oral, or dermal) and can be classified according to systemic, immunologic, neurologic, reproductive, developmental, or carcinogenic effects following acute (14 days or less), intermediate (15–364 days), and chronic (365 days or more) exposure periods. Based on studies of nickel workers and laboratory animals, all nickel compounds, except for metallic nickel, have been classified as human carcinogens by the International agency for research on cancer (IARC).

HEAVY METALS AS FREE RADICAL GENERATORS

The mechanisms of heavy metals toxicity through electron transfer most often involve the cross linking of the sulfhydryl groups of proteins. Nickel and other heavy metals can also generate free radicals directly from molecular oxygen in a two step process to produce superoxide anion. In the continued presence of the heavy metal, the superoxide anions formed can then combine with protons in the dismutation reaction generating hydrogen peroxide in the process. Although, nickel (II) by itself does not cause efficient free radical generation from oxygen, H_2O_2, or lipid hydroperoxides, the reactivity of Ni (II) with those oxygen derivatives can be modulated by chelation with certain histidine- and cysteine-containing ligands. The incubation of Ni (II) with cysteine in an aerobic environment generates the hydroxyl radical, which then reacts with cysteine to generate a carbon-centered alkyl radical[5]. Free radicals can also be generated from lipid hydroperoxides by Ni (II) in the presence of several oligopeptides.

NICKEL ON HEALTH

In acute toxicity of nickel, there is report of a rise in blood insulin level, a profound increase in serum prolactin level, alteration of several enzymatic activities and respiratory tract problem[6,7,8]. Gastroenteritis, nausea, vomiting, tremor, diarrhea, nasal secretion, itching, dyspnea and dry cough are the symptoms observed after acute nickel toxicity[9]. Chronic exposure to different nickel compounds leads to irreversible lung damage, abnormal pulmonary functions, renal tubular necrosis, anemia, eosinophilia, nasal septum ulceration, allergic dermatitis, finally leading to cancer[10]. Reports were also available of decreased sperm count and motility along with suppression of testicular steroidogenic enzymes after intermediary nickel exposure[11]. Chronic toxicity induced decreased protein synthesis, inhibition of ATPase activity leading to neurological disorders. Some of the recent studies done by this laboratory revealed that nickel sulfate has reversible degenerative effect on hepatic tissues of rat and alter the serum lipid profile. Increased lipid peroxide level along with decreased activity of various antioxidant enzymes in various metabolically active tissues in rats were also noticed[12,13]. Similar observation was also found in case of erythrocyte antioxidant enzyme status[14].

ANTIOXIDANT DEFENSE

Suitable mechanisms are there in our body so that steady state concentration of potentially toxic oxygen derived free radicals are kept in check under normal physiological condition by body's intrinsic antioxidant defense system, but enhanced generation of these reactive oxygen species (ROS) can overwhelm cell's intrinsic antioxidant defenses and result in a condition known as "oxidative stress". Data suggests that antioxidants may play an important role in abating some hazards of nickel[15]. Exogenous antioxidants are intimately involved in the prevention of cellular damage by interacting with free radicals and by terminating the chain reaction. In rats, increased lipid peroxide formation and decreased levels of glutathione, SOD, CAT, GSH-Px activities as well as ascorbic acid depletion have been found in the most active metabolic tissues of the body, namely, liver and kidney [12, 16]. Increased lipid peroxidation could stimulate phospholipase A_2 (PLA_2) activities, thereby causing the production of a variety of eicosanoids, products of the arachidonic acid pathway that are responsible for cell injury. Additionally, a decrease in antioxidant enzymes suggests an interaction with the accumulated free radicals and active amino acids of the enzymes, leading to functional impairment and tissue damage. Ascorbic acid (Vitamin C) is a dietary antioxidant that inactivates oxygen free radicals. Some studies have shown that vitamin C works in concert with vitamin E to prevent the free radical chain oxidation of lipids. Numerous reports have shown the positive effect of vitamin C as an antioxidant and scavenger of free radicals. Nickel compounds adversely affect cells by modulating ascorbic-acid metabolism and other metabolic pathways. Reports have shown the positive effect of vitamin C as an antioxidant and scavenger of free radicals. On the other hand, doses of Vitamin C exceeding the daily recommended dietary allowance could lead to the formation of toxic advanced glycation end products, which are derived from the degradation products of carbohydrates, lipids, and ascorbic acid.

Numerous animal studies support the ability of vitamin C to protect against free radical damage in vitro. One of our study revealed that, L-ascorbic administration simultaneously with nickel sulfate improve nickel induced hyperglycemia by boosting insulin sensitivity in rats and also improve liver glycogen content[17]. The administration of L-ascorbic acid can improve the situation in rats by its scavenging activity within the lipid region of the membrane. Reports also showed that both the nickel-induced activation of hypoxia-inducible factor (HIF-1) and the upregulation of hypoxia-inducible genes are due to depleted intracellular ascorbate levels. The addition of ascorbate to the culture medium increased the intracellular ascorbate level and reversed both the metal-induced stabilization of HIF-1 and HIF-1α dependent gene expression[18]. α- tocopherol (Vitamin E) can also protect against oxidative stress and improve nickel induced alteration of serum lipid profile and plasma glucose concentration. It is also reported that, α- tocopherol can protect both liver and pancreatic cells from nickel induced cellular damage[17]. Vitamin E, situated near the cytochrome P-450 in the membrane phospholipid, sweeps the free radicals formed in the cytochrome P-450.

CONCLUSION

We can conclude from the various studies cited, including those conducted by the present author and his group, that nickel is a potent hematotoxic, hepatotoxic, pulmonary toxic, and nephrotoxic agent. Although conflicting results have been reported in human studies of the effect of L-ascorbic acid and alpha-tocopherol supplementation on oxidative stress, the experimental animal results with ascorbic acid suggest that a high consumption of dietary L-ascorbic acid and α-tocopherol might ameliorate nickel-induced oxidative stress.

Acknowledgement

The authors greatly acknowledge the Ditector, Defence Institute of Physiology and Allied Sciences, New Delhi (DRDO, Ministry of Defence, Government of India) for providing financial assistance (*Ref.No. TC/ 260/ TASK-91 (KKD)/ DIPAS/ 2004 dt.07.06.2004*)

References

1. Agency for Toxic Substances and Disease Registry (ATSDR). Toxicological Profile for Nickel. U.S. Department of Health and Human Services, Public Health Service, ATSDR. Atlanta, Georgia, USA: U.S. Government Printing Office 2003; 5–16.

2. Sunderman FW Jr. Sources of exposure and biological effects of nickel. In: O'Neill IK, Schuller P, Fishbein L, eds. Environmental carcinogens selected methods of analysis. Volume 8: Some metals: As, Be, Cd, Cr, Ni, Pb, Se, Zn. IARC scientific publication no. 71. Lyon, France: Internation Agency for Research on Cancer 1986; 79-92

3. Scansetti G, Maina G, Botta GC, Bambace P, Spinelli P. Exposure to cobalt and nickel in the hard metal production industry. *Int Arch Occup Environ Health* 1998; 71: 60–63.

4. Angerer J, Lehnert G. Occupational chronic exposure to metals. II: Nickel exposure of stainless steel welders – biological monitoring. *Int Arch Occup Environ Health* 1990; 62: 7-10

5. Shi X, Dalal NS, Kasprzak KS. Generation of free radicals in reaction of Ni(II)-thiol complexes with molecular oxygen and model lipid hydroperoxides. *J.Inorg.Biochem* 1993, 50(3): 211-225

6. Sunderman FW, Kincaid JF. Nickel poisoning. II. Studies on patients suffering from acute exposure to vapors of nickel carbonyl. *J Am Med Assoc.* 1954; 155(10): 889-94.

7. Clemons G, Garcia JF. Neuroendocrine effects of acute nickel chloride administration in rats. *Toxicol Appl Pharmacol* 1981; 61 (3): 343-348

8. Sanfold WE, Neiboer E, Bach P, Stace B, Gregg N, Dobrota N. The renal clearance & toxicity of nickel. In: 4th International Conference on Nockel Metabolism & Toxicology, abstracts, Espoo, Finland, 5 – 9 Sep, Helsinki Institute of Occupational Health 1988; p 17

9. Sunderman FW Jr, Coulston F, Eichhorn GL. Nickel. Washington DC, National Academy of Science 1975; 97-143

10. Nielsen FH. Possible future implications of nickel, arsenic, silicon, vanadium and other ultra trace elements in human nutrition. In: Clinical and biochemical nutritional aspects of trace elements. New York, NY: Alan R. Liss Inc 1982; 379-404.

11. Das KK, Dasgupta S. Effect of nickel sulfate on testicular steroidogenesis in rats during protein restriction. *Environ Health Perspect* 2002; 110 (9): 923–926.

12. Das KK, Gupta AD, Dhundasi SA, et al. Effect of L-ascorbic acid on nickel-induced alterations in serum lipid profiles and liver histopathology of rats. *J Basic Clin Physiol Pharmacol* 2006; 17 (1): 29–44.

13. Gupta, AD, Patil AM, Ambekar JG, Das SN, Dhundasi SA & Das KK (2006). L-ascorbic acid protects the antioxidant defense system in nickel-exposed albino rat lung tissues. *J Basic Clin Physiol Pharmacol*, 17(2), 87-100

14. Das KK, Gupta AD, Dhundasi SA, Patil AM, Das SN, Ambekar JG. Protective Role of L-ascorbic acid on antioxidant defense system in erythrocytes of albino rats exposed to nickel sulfate. *Biometals.* 2007;20(2): 177-84.

15. Ercal N, Gurer-Orhan H, Aykin-Burns N. Toxic metals and oxidative stress part I: mechanisms involved in metal induced oxidative damage. *Curr Top Med Chem* 2001; 1: 529-539

16. Das KK, Dasgupta S. Studies on the role of nickel in the metabolism of ascorbic acid and cholesterol in experimental animals. Ind J Physiol Allied Sci 1998; 52 (2): 58–62.

17. Das KK. Project report submitted to DIPAS, DRDO, Delhi. Ministry of Defence, Government of India, 2006; Ref. No.TC/260/TASK-91(KKD)/DIPAS/2004 Dated 07/06/2004).

18. Salnikow K, Donald SP, Bruick RK, Zhitkovich A, Phang JM, Kasprzak KS. Depletion of intracellular ascorbate by the carcinogenic metal nickel and cobalt results in the induction of hypoxic stress. *J Biol Chem* 2004, 279, 40337-40344

19. Das KK, Buchner V. Effect of Nickel Exposure on Peripheral Tissues: Role of Oxidative Stress in Toxicity and Possible Protection by Ascorbic Acid. *Rev Environ Health* 2007, 22(2): 133-149

7

Seat-desk: Some Ergonomic Design Concerns

Debkumar Chakrabarti

Department of Design, Indian Institute of Technology Guwahati
Guwahati 781 039

ABSTRACT

Ergonomics has advanced its design applications from machine dominance to usability and pleasure while interacting with product to ensure joy in use. User analyses product's attributes through knowing, doing and feeling which is linked with his cognitive skills, perceptual-motor skills and emotional skills. Design ergonomics plays role in addressing criteria for good human compatible and context specific design including body support devices. Recent experiments advocate a shift from confined work posture to flexible posture adopted work culture, and accordingly studies to appropriate context specific ways and means to achieve that is now a research focus by many concerns. A good design creates a context for experience that fully respects user's all inbuilt capabilities and acquired skills, and understands users and their requirements. It aids human functional needs as well as pleasure whereas an inappropriate design induces stress, and improper use and misuse appears as trouble makers.

Seating is a diverse activity in the simple sense that there can be infinitely many ways of sitting for different people and many times may involve different people sitting in different postures doing the same activity. This paper focuses application of ergonomics principles and criteria for seated work and emphasises use context and anthropometric considerations of seat and work desk design. Some design concepts have been conceived in order to ensure flexibility in movement, comfortable posture and better performance. These include design and development of (1) a personal computer table for general use, (2) seat-desk combined unit for class room use in school by children, (3) a separate unit of a height adjustable drawing table and semi-sitting multi functional high stool for engineering drafting purpose which is being used by IIT Guwahati students and (4) a concept for mobile lecture delivery with computer and LCD projection assistance. These designs satisfy dimensional compatibility between users' body geometry and cognitive aspects of specific task needs and design features, and above all it sees aspects of pleasure beyond functionality as an immerging issue in seating design.

1.0 AESTHETIC UTILITY AND TRUST IN DESIGN

Ergonomics has advanced its design applications from machine dominance to usability and pleasure while interacting with products to ensure joy in use. User analyses product's attributes through knowing, doing and feeling which is linked with his cognitive skills, perceptual-motor skills and emotional skills. Application of best scientific principles and appropriate technologies may generate a design best to deliver its intended function, still its user, the prime system component, ultimately has to feel comfort while using it to qualify the same a good design.

Design is an innovative, practical, reproducible solution to conceive various aids to human needs. It is a continuous problem solving process with conversion of ideas into reality, keeping in minds the user's characteristics and limitations, art and aesthetics, material and process, and new technology. Good designs thus follow human, inbuilt as well as acquired, abilities and limitations in terms of physical, physiological and behavioral aspects.

Design ergonomics plays role in addressing criteria for good human compatible and context specific design including body support devices. Recent experiments advocate a shift from confined work posture to flexible posture adopted work culture, and accordingly studies to appropriate context specific ways and means to achieve that is now a research focus by many concerns. A good design creates a context for experience that fully respects user's all inbuilt capabilities and acquired skills, and understands users and their requirements, Fig. 1. It aids human functional needs as well as pleasure to use and possess. A good design reduces stress through appropriate use of usability elements. Though a design is conceived with all good features, improper use and misuse appears as trouble makers. The issue is how we see these in design application; design should be human compatible and context specific.

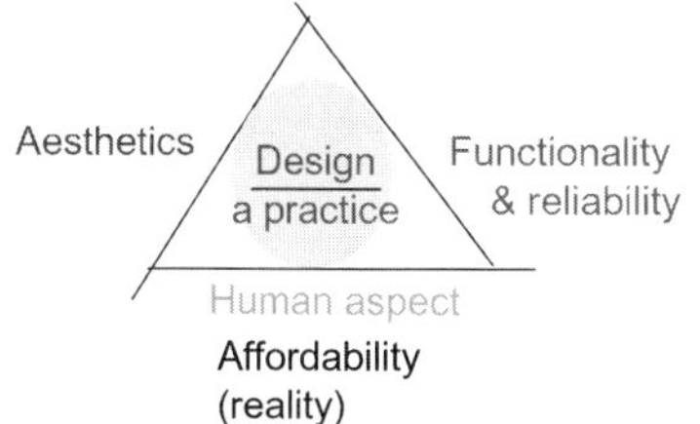

Fig. 1 Factors responsible for humanising design.

Product Ergonomics optimises the functionality, safety and comfort of products, especially when the physical interaction between man, product and surroundings is intensive. It requires design features and human functional need match, and perceptual bias and its relation to our aesthetic preferences in man made world as well as in nature. Design with organic form creates mildness in appearance.

2.0 SOME ASPECTS OF ERGONOMICS FOR CONCEIVING SEAT-DESK DEVICES

Among various design applications, role of ergonomics dealing with furniture and body supportive devices for various purposes appears to be predominant. Seating is a diverse activity in the simple sense that there can be infinitely many ways of sitting for different people and many times may involve different people sitting in different postures doing the same activity. This paper focuses application of ergonomics principles and criteria for sitstand work, emphasises use context and users information. Commercial advertisements also uses ergonomics as value added terms to express more comfort in use and safety is being used as commercial benefit. Ergonomics has become a business promotion word that we hear so often these days, particularly in the high-tech industry tagged to their products. Ergonomics is a way to work smarter and not harder, and it can be achieved by designing tools, equipment, work stations to suit intended tasks as well as leisure time requirements.

While talking about human benefits and limitations, and its seat-desk design relevance along with human movement and circulation in a work space, the below is a must to consider:

- Man occupies a specific space of his own body form-size-shape and when he moves the space also moves.
- When he adopts different postures, the same body space changes accordingly.
- Differences between space occupied by an inanimate object and the man are that the human space is not only fixed (which the body physically occupies) but it needs some additional space as psychological territory feeling and this varies from task to task, even person to person, and also differs according to body proportions of an individual.
- This additional space requirement is clearances.
- Children adopt free postures and at the increment of age compromising with surroundings and adapting to various tasks situations our posture and movement becomes constrained; and at the same time our body looses flexibility and become more rigid. Body growth and behaviour adaptation must be considered while conceiving a design for body support and work with.

The issue is how we see design application of the above to get maximum benefit; design should be human compatible and context specific, and to reach the goal the below mentioned aspects may be considered:

- Varieties of postures are used in daily activities, which need task and context specific design considerations. Product and space features to deliver intended function should match with user's capabilities and should be context specific; Psychological factors e.g., mood, emotion etc., influences product features. We perform tasks also that quite often adopt awkward posture and impose ergonomics risks. Taking into account of the triangle of ergonomics risk factors, which comprises posture, frequency and force, design should take care if any one is ease out, it would minimise the risk.

- Work environment consists of work furniture and work equipment; while use these work furniture, work equipment and machines in various work settings we experience varieties of postural constraints. Design of these products and their layout in workspace would be inviting if it provides free posture adoption facility at users own will. Today's office work environment is experiencing a shift from formal to semiformal approach. This opens up challenges to make new work places and functional furniture support.

- Design support to defend a specific task demanding posture needs to be justified. Furniture support must match functional requirements and operation easiness; obstacles while reaching to the work component and physical mismatch results in uneasiness. A large portion of time we spent using seat-desk posture; thus attention has also to be given to work surface area, location and tilt in respect to the user in seated as well as standing posture

- Product geometry and user's anthropometry (both in static as well as dynamic considerations of use) should complement each other to ensure safety as well as better function. Some ergonomics consideration addresses these issues
  - o Anthropometric dimensions (Indian data for Indian use must be considered):
    - Static human body dimensions are used initial stages of design development to conceptualise the design, and
    - Dynamic dimensions considering task demanding body movement are necessary to finalise the design dimensions to match different task performances and during leisure time,
  - o Behaviour: to fit the dimensions with cognitive issues of intended users, and,
  - o Physiological: ensure safe limits while using the design.
- Seat-desk design must confirm:
  - o Parallel relationship between trunk and shank;
  - o The heights of the work surface, seat and feet position must be compatible;

- o Ensure barrier less free leg room and a footrest if the work height is fixed;
- o Work platform heights and slants vary with the nature of tasks performed;
- o Workstation layout and horizontal work zones along with arm arc distances;
- o Front working space clearance should be in line with the primary work zone;
- o Arm rest support depending on task requirement may be extended from the working surface.
- Organic appearance in recent design application ensures mild and pleasant look to the product that can be used in seat-desk design whereas with conventional application of strong straight lines and sharp angles produce visual rigidity.

3.0 SOME DESIGN CONCEPTS ADDRESSING CONTEXT SPECIFIC ISSUES

Design is normally created out of local needs, and thus carries an identity. Such some design concepts have been conceived in order to ensure flexibility in movement, comfortable posture and better performance. Below are four concepts that have been developed in tune to the above mentions:

3.1 Simplicity in Design: A Table that can Also be Used as Personal Computer Worktable

A concept for a multipurpose table, with two platforms, top one to be used as main work surface and bottom one as footrest and for occasional storage, mainly for single person's use where two persons can also work together, was carried out, Fig. 2. This study was done to see if the simple form of a table can perform tasks with computer without any special keyboard-mouse drawer fitted under the top work surface. Many workstation designs with various attachments and keyboard-mouse drawer are available in market and acclaimed to be ergonomic computer table. It is also observed that improper use of keyboard drawer dimensions induces restriction to the hand and body movement. Inappropriate use of the product away from its intended use mode and products designed without considering users' compatibility features lacks in product reliability and safety which finally land to be trouble makers.

Objectives of this study was to see if simple designed table with dimensions concerning various human movement can perform the similar task with all the necessary equipment placed within the structure as well as this can also be used for other purposes for general tasks; for computer work only perhaps a separate complex design items is not necessary as a compulsion. This table was expected to be used as an additional table in small hostel rooms where compute work can also be done. Trial results (students of IIT Guwahati) show simplicity approach provides more freeness in the context of 'as and whenever required to be used'; design features conceived to provide better functionality such as provision of keyboard-mouse drawer and concealed wiring system, etc., sometimes restrict movement and confines the posture while doing certain task. Keyboard, mouse, monitor, scanner, printer and other accessories, e.g., paper holders, etc., are to be placed within various arm reach zones without any visual as well as physical obstacle to get reach to the without changing body positions. For development of a furniture item it requires to identify the support features for the basic need and simplicity in structure, and the design should be constraints free as far as possible.

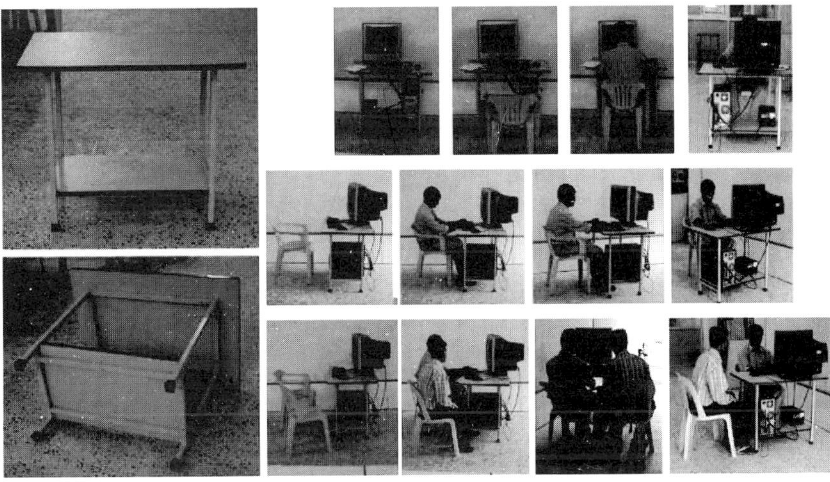

Fig. 2 Simple concept of a table with two layer platform, the top one to be used as main work surface and bottom one for other storage as well as can also be used as footrest. Product dimensions follow the ease of user's body parts movement while work with computer.

3.2 A Seat-desk Combined Unit for Class Room Use in School by Children

A new classroom combined seat-desk unit, Fig. 3, for age group 6-8 years, students' of 1st to 3rd standard was developed. Special considerations were taken not only on the users' (Indian Children) body dimensions but particular behaviour of the users; they require sitting, reading and writing, standing in between seat and desk, and the structure should be sturdy enough to absorb the shock from students' mischievous behaviour. While conceiving design dimensions trials, Fig. 4, with likely to be users have been taken into account.

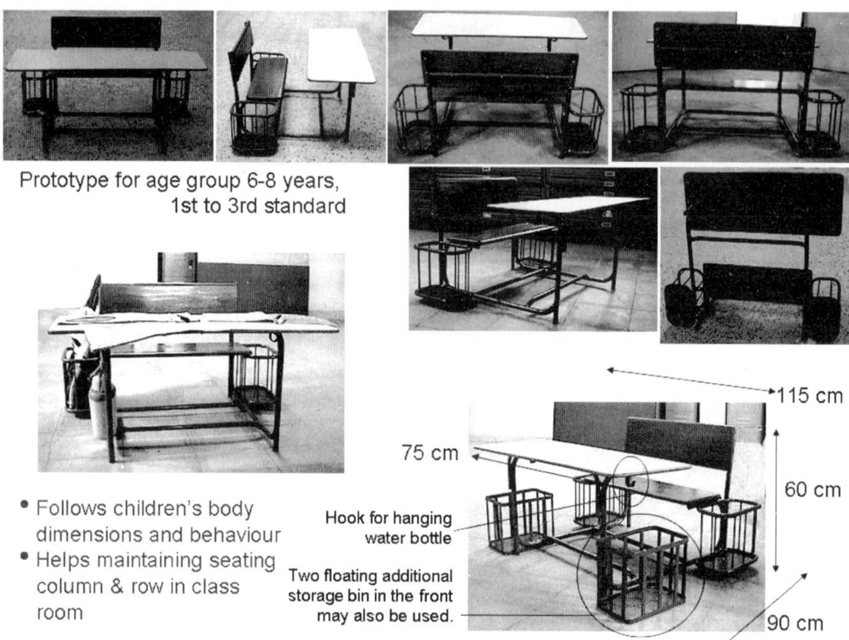

Fig. 3 A concept for classroom seat-desk device, for age group 6-8 years, Students' of 1st to 3rd standard.

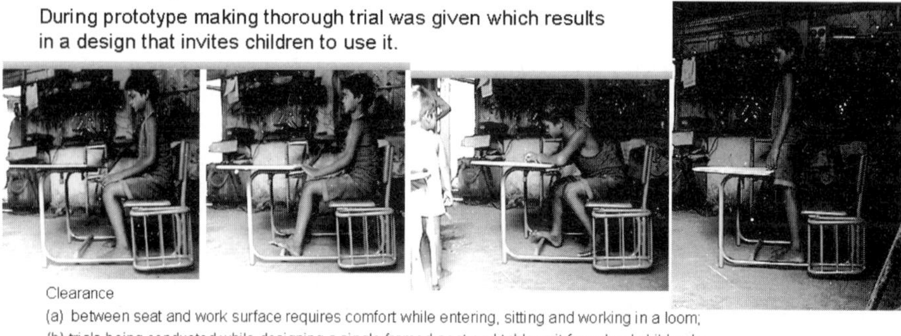

Clearance
(a) between seat and work surface requires comfort while entering, sitting and working in a loom;
(b) trials being conducted while designing a single framed seat and table unit for school children's
use which requires occasionally standing and also provides easiness in getting in and out.

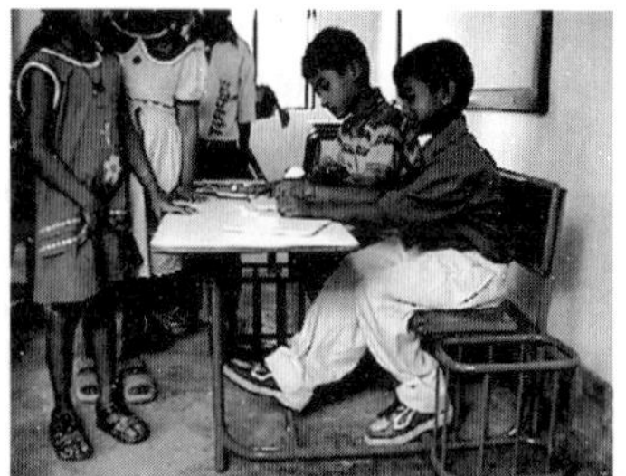

- This simple design can be mass-produced (even by local artisans) and it is not only durable, but any damaged part can also be replaced without disturbing other components, and is easy to maintain.

- The design goes in tune with the playful nature of children, confirms the ergonomic concept of fitting the design to children and the task, and provides greater comfort.

- Such look good and work good furniture would promote an atmosphere more conducive to the learning process.

Fig. 4 Clearances between seat and desk have been made through trial results.

3.3 DRAWING TABLE AND STOOL WITH SIT-STAND POSTURE REQUIREMENT

A high stool for multi-posture adoption facility with three different height tying members on the legs has been conceived with hip rest as basic concept, Fig. 5.

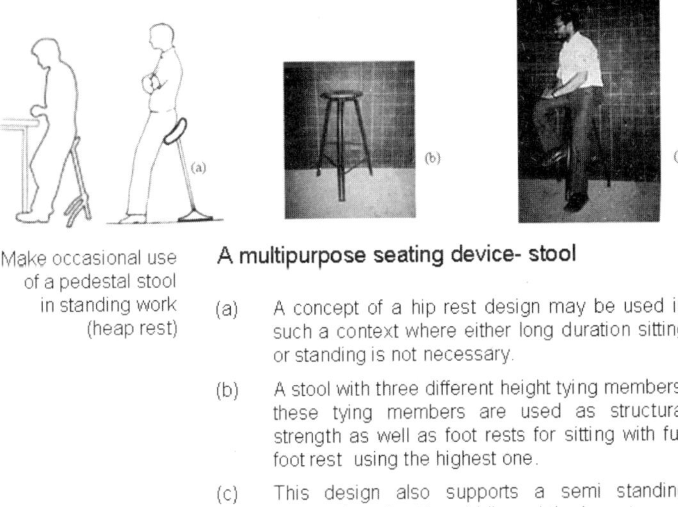

Fig. 5 A high seat with hip rest concept.

A unit of an angle adjustable drawing table and a semi-sitting multi functional high stool (based on the above hip rest concept), Fig. 6, was developed with wood top and metal frame for students undergoing higher

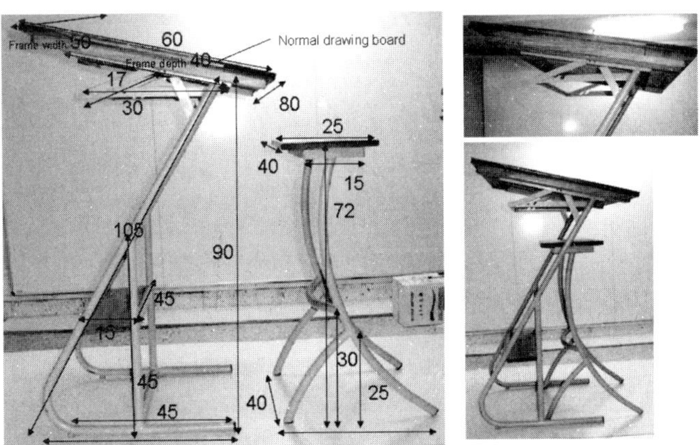

Fig. 6 An angle adjustable engineering drawing table and high stool unit.

studies at IIT Guwahati. Dimensions and ranges of adjustability have been identified after analysing the task needs by the students for drafting engineering drawing. A number of such units are in use at engineering drawing studio of IIT Guwahati. This unit not only satisfy the task need, look-wise it is aesthetic; its overall appearance can be classified as 'satisfying aesthetic functionality'.

3.4 SLICK MOBILE LECTURE DELIVERY ASSISTANCE DEVICE

A concept for mobile lecture delivery assistance, Fig. 7, (with computer etc., modern facilities, to suit ceiling mounted LCD projection, inbuilt multiple power points, four rotating wheels with stoppers, foot rest, push-pull horizontal handle, etc features) was developed.

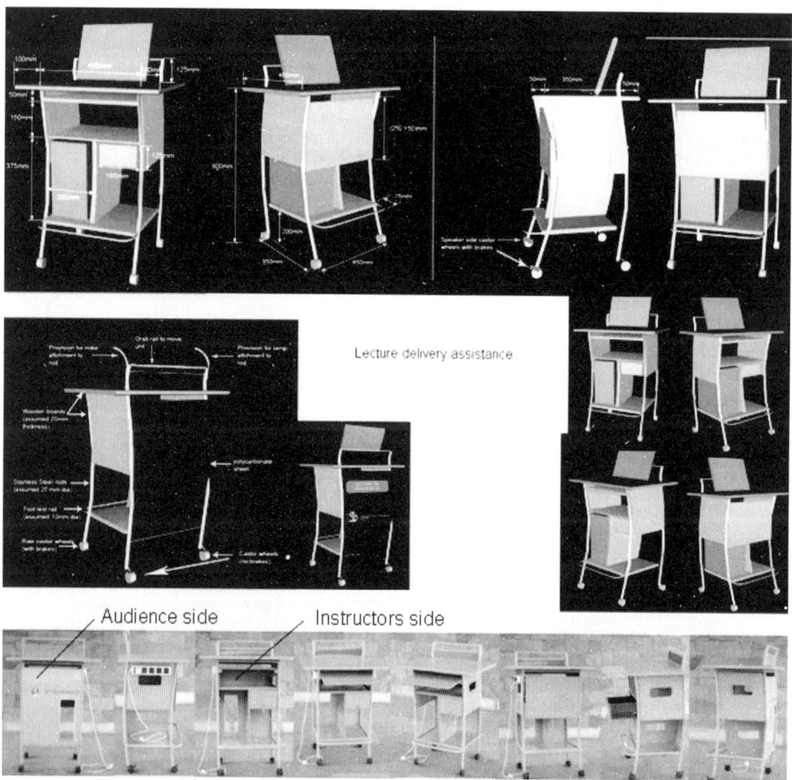

Fig. 7 Mobile (on the dais) lecture delivery assistance with organic look- a concept.

This design satisfies the dimensional compatibility between users' body geometry and cognitive aspects of specific task needs, i.e., the delivery of lecture in a class room or in an auditorium. Specific compartments are devoted to be used as storage for various accessory items. It has an extendable plate under the table top that can be used when pulled out as an extension of the top table surface as well as when it is lowered down to the front it can cover the drawer and lock the compartments. Approach of using organic form with mild curvatures ensures pleasing look.

4.0 CONCLUSION

Every product we use, it may be a utility consumer product, a furniture item or a workspace layout, we are always judging its acceptance value asking exactly what it is and how it looks (form), what it does (function), and how it performs (linking this two with human compatibility); and above all it sees aspects of pleasure beyond functionality which today is an immerging issue in the field of design ergonomics.

Design features are not only to divulge ease of use and safety the functional needs but pleasure of use, enjoyment of the experience; it should be aesthetically appealing and dimensions matching with users' features.

References

Banerjee, S., Goel, K.M., Chakrabarti, D. and Das, A. 2006: An Approach to Specify Informal

Chakrabarti, D. 1997: Indian Anthropometric dimensions for ergonomic design practice; ISBN No: 81-86199-15-0, 161p, published in 1997 by National Institute of Design, Paldi, Ahmedabad 380007

Chakrabarti, D. 2001: Design Ergonomics: Need and Role, Special issue on ergonomics & Human Factors engineering, ISSN 0970-3365, Udyog Pragati, the journal for Practicing Managers, National Institute of Industrial Engineering, Mumbai- 400087, India, April-June, 25:2, Pp. 37-43.

Chakrabarti, D. 2005: Ergonomics/Human Factors: Human aspect of Technology, Directions,

Chakrabarti, D. 2006: Product Ergonomics, Indo-US Design Workshop, January, IISc, Bangalore.

Chakrabarti, D. 2007: Anthropometry and Some Design Issues, in "Ergonomic Interventions for Health & Productivity' edited by Dr. (Mrs.) Suman Singh (Maharana Pratap University of Agriculture & Technology), Himanshu Publications, Daryaganj, New Delhi.

Chakrabarti, D. 2007: Role of Ergonomics in Making Consumer Products Usable and Pleasurable, International Conference on Frontier researches in Integrative Physiology (ICFRIP), Kolkata, 2007, January 8-10.

Chakrabarti, D. and Das, A. 2004: Design Development of a New Seat-desk Unit Suitable for Indian School Children, Proc. National Conference on Humanising Work and Work Environment, April , 22- 24, 2004, TIFAC-CORE NITIE, National Institute of Industrial Engineering, Mumbai, Pp. 131-136.

Chakrabarti, D. and Nag, P.K. 1996: Human concept in workspace design, Ergonomics and work design- emerging issues in organisational sciences, ISBN 81-224-0865-6, New age international (P) ltd., New Delhi, India, Pp. 129-156.

Das, A. and Chakrabarti, D. 2004: Role of free postural adoption on performance and informal workplace design, Proc. National Conference on Humanising Work and Work Environment, April, 22-24, 2004, TIFAC-CORE NITIE., National Institute of Industrial Engineering, Mumbai, Pp. 72-76.

Indian Institute of Technology Kanpur, Vol. 7, Issue 1 March, Special Issue on Product Design and Media Communication, Pp. 41-47.

International Ergonomics Conference) December 10-12, 2005, ISBN 81-8424-124-0, Allied Publishers Pvt., Ltd., New Delhi, Pp. 144-148.

Sitting in Classroom, Proceedings HWWE2005 (Humanizing Work and Work Environment,

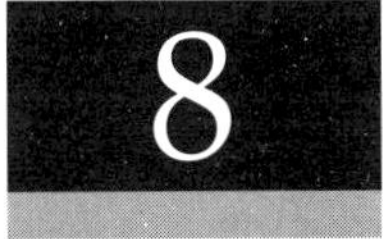

Ergonomics in Sports – Indian Context

Asis Goswami

Ex. Senior Scientific Officer, SAI
96 Ruby Park East, Kolkata – 700078

ABSTRACT

Application of ergonomics in sports has been happening for quite some time. However, in absence of a defined boundary it is difficult to include or omit published article from the limits of review. The present review has made an attempt to find the starting point in ergonomics application in sports. The review has arranged articles in series of decades till 2005. It was found that there is decline in the number of sports ergonomics publications in the new millennium.

INTRODUCTION

Ergonomics is a relatively new discipline of science & technology. Since beginning of the specialized area of knowledge "Ergonomics" there were focused effort to obtain a balance in Man-Machine-Environment. Slowly "Ergonomics concepts" made its inroad to industry, defence, home, in all aspects of life. However, entry of ergonomics in sports is a delayed response, until "sports" became an industry itself.

1.0 WHAT SHOULD BE CONSIDERED AS SPORTS ERGONOMICS WORK? AN ISSUE YET TO BE RESOLVED

During the inception of the concept "Ergonomics" K.F.H. Murrell had defined the special area as "the study of the relationship between man and his working environment" (Murrell, 1960). In 1983 the editorial in Ergonomics journal expressed "The strength of ergonomics is that it does not consider the findings from one discipline to be an irrelevance to the conclusions drawn from another; it is the interaction between the disciplines that makes ergonomics."

Ergonomics is a multidisciplinary approach and has a wide application to everyday situations in any kind of work place. It has significant implications for efficiency, productivity, safety and health in work settings. The ergonomics specialist is expected to work in teams that may involve a variety of other professions that include physiologists, psychologists, design engineers, production engineers, industrial designers, computer specialists, industrial physicians, health and safety practitioners, and the like. However the focus remains at most productive use of human capabilities, and the maintenance of human health and well-being. The definition and approach had radical changes with more people from diverse discipline entered in Ergonomics. In an effort to resolve the ambiguity in the terminology the *International Ergonomics Association* had adopted the following definition in August 2000:

"Ergonomics (or human factors) is the scientific discipline concerned with the understanding of interactions among humans and other elements of a system, and the profession that applies theory, principles, data, and other methods to design in order to optimize human well-being and overall system performance."

One may argue that a research work focused to "removal mechanism of blood lactate" also contributes to a better understanding of system performance and hence should be considered as ergonomics study. Considering this argument any work or activity related to sports can be classified as "Sports Ergonomics" study. Such a condition would lead to confusion in the long term and the discipline "Ergonomics" will loose its characteristics. Two important characteristics distinguish the subject from others and they are 1) multidisciplinary approach and 2) application of knowledge to improve system performance. It is obligatory to distinguish between research activities and the activities that would characterize and influence practitioners. In one article J.P. Clarys expressed that an ergonomist may base his analysis or recommendation on the results of basic research and this may be a prerequisite for an ergonomist. However, the scientist at the basic research end may not target his research to solve an ergonomics problem (Clarys, 1988).

Similar approach was also taken by many sports scientists in Germany and USA in the form of 'Sports Medicine'. The focus had significant difference. Sports Medicine had medical orientation of the approach in contrast to engineering & design approach in sports ergonomics. A detail discussion on this issue could be found in the article by Goswami (2001). Probably overlapping of scientific work sometimes makes discipline wise differences indistinguishable.

A full review of the historical developments is not the aim of this document. However, some review is provided below to help understanding of the concepts and future demand. A literature survey was made and articles with classical ergonomics approach are discussed below:

2.0   A LOOK AT THE PUBLISHED LITERATURE

2.1   Early Developments (1980-1989)

It is difficult to find a date for beginning of ergonomics application in sports. First ever publication could be traced to 1981. Reilly (1981) wrote about the inflexibility of demand in sports and need for interdisciplinary approach to estimate the task demand. Application of ergonomics in design of sports equipment and facility was also advocated.

In 1983 **Catalano and Hanccock** presented a review on Human factors of Sport during 27th Annual Meeting of Human Factors Society at Norfolk, Virginia. Some studies related to sports ergonomics were underway at John Moores University, Liverpool, UK, during the same period.

Articles directly related to sports ergonomics started appearing in Ergonomics journals as early as 1984. In this year the journal "Applied Ergonomics" had published a number of articles in the specialized area. It was emphasized that most of the methodologies applied in industrial ergonomics has relevance to studies of ergonomics in sports (Reilly, 1984). There is no doubt that "Time and Motion study" used in industrial 'work study' is of immense potential in analysis of matches in sports. Atha (1984) highlighted the developments in motion analysis during that period and its use sports. Renewed interest of The Ergonomics society in sports and fitness led to the First international Conference on Sport, Leisure and Ergonomics in 1987. The proceedings was published in a special issue of Ergonomics in 1988 (November). The movement took momentum and the conference became a feature in every three years. The sports ergonomics we see at present is the result of this major effort.

Importance of ergonomics in sports equipment design was clearly indicated by Reilly and Lees (1984). Sports equipments could be categorized as 1) equipment used for specific sport; 2) those used during training and 3) ergometers for evaluation of performance capacities. In many cases ergometers can be sport specific and serve dual purpose of evaluation and training. Tennis racquet and synthetic playing surface are examples of the first category. Safety, specificity and design were key ergonomic issues raised in relation to matching sports person with the sporting environment. Possible ergonomics intervention in officiating and spectating at sporting events was also indicated. Safety and performance were also ergonomics issues dealt by Fredrick (1984) in relation to shoe design. Damaging effect of boxing punch and its biomechanical characteristics was also investigated (Atha, 1985). Safety aspects of synthetic surfaces was studied in two sports : football and tennis (Nigg & Segesser, 1988).

It was interesting that during the early development of sports ergonomics computer application possibility was also explored (Lees, 1985). Leaving no stones unturned Clarys (1985) attempted to search ergonomics links in swimming. It involved study of hydrodynamics, applied dynamics of swimming, electromyography and training aspects. Alternative training systems was recommended. Role of electromyography in sports ergonomics was studied in greater detail in a later publication also (Clarys et al, 1988). Computerized notation analysis was employed successfully by Hughes (1988) in field games analysis. Time motion analysis of handball game was carried out by a Canadian Group. Work rest ratio in handball was found to be 1:1 and training suggestion was provided on the basis of observations of the study. (Alexander & Boreskie, 1989).

One of the dark sides of ergonomics application is increased comfort and inactivity. Optimization of work lead to reduced energy expenditure. Well designed work process would increase repetitive low demand tasks. With this speculation Shephard (1988) highlighted the need for ergonomics inputs in designing leisure and sports activity in the industry as well as outside.

2.2 The Nineties (1990-1999)

Last decade of the 21st Century witnessed proliferation of research activities in sports and ergonomics. Indian contribution to sports ergonomics started during this period.

Computer simulation of sports skill was attempted by Yeadon et al (1990). The difference between computer simulation based on anthropometric measurements and actual skill performance (airborne phase of somersault) was found to be small. The difference could be explained from the error in anthropometric measurement or film digitization errors. One of the important determinants of success in archery is thought to be postural consistency. On the contrary large variability in precision in the pre-loose stance of the archers was observed and a doubt was raised about the usability of video analysis for elite level archers (Stuart & Atha, 1990). Detail examination of badminton shuttlecock was made by Alison J. Cooke (1992) which led to the marketing of new variety of aerodynamically designed shuttlecocks.

International Symposium on Ergonomics, Occupational Health, Safety and Environment was held at IIT, Bombay (Jan. 2 6) which had presentations on sports ergonomics. This was the first official recognition of sports ergonomics in India. Posture analysis was also attempted by Goswami et al (1991). They estimated the distance covered by a badminton player during competitive matches using "String diagram" method that is conventionally used in work study. Same study did also try to use the posture targeting method (described by Corlett et al (19)) to reach an understanding about the postural stress among badminton players. Attempt was also made to analyse hockey matches using similar method after recording the matches in video (Thapliwal, 1991).

In 1991 Applied Ergonomics published again a collection of papers on sports ergonomics. The papers gave a feel of the classical ergonomics methodologies in the environment of sports and physical activity (Reilly, 1991a 1991b; Davids, 1991). In the same year 2nd Interantional Conference was held with greater support from different sporting associations. Selected papers were published in Ergonomics (1994). By this time technology transfer from industry to sports began to take place. Portable oxygen analyzer was a long pending requirement in field evaluation of sports activities and a portable analyzer was also evaluated (Forkink and Frings-Dresen, 1994). One equipment V-scope is an essential part of training for Olympic weight lifting at present had roots in the application for occupational manual material handling and clinical exercise therapy (Charteris et al, 1994). Learning of motor skills is common for both industry and sports. A thorough study was presented by Annet (1994) encompassing both these aspects. Tactical analysis could be achived through motion analysis of a particular player and this was shown by the experiments of Hughes & Franks (1994). They observed that significant differences in all the velocities and the accelerations between the winning rallies and losing rallies are present between Elite and Provincial groups (p < 0.10). It explained the basis for a tactical approach to attempt to reduce the opponents' playing time by taking the ball as early as possible. Similar attempt was made by Hong et al (1996) using notational systems. Safety aspects and injury prevention was considered in cycling with prediction of optimal posture (de Vey Mestdagh, 1998). Women participants in sports face unique challenge due to their feminine features. Displacement of breast can be large enough to cause pain. Good designs of brassiere could prevent such conditions (Page & Steele, 1999).

One of the significant developments of the last decade was formation of International Sports Engineering Association in 1998 at in Sheffield (UK). The association aims to act as a forum for discussion on technical and scientific issues relating to sport and sport technology. ISEA has been publishing the International Sports Engineering Journal since 1998. Establishment of ISEA and the publication of journal created fresh impetus in the developments that was gathering momentum.

2.3 THE NEW MILLENNIUM (2000-2005)

A three dimensional regression model of shoulder was developed by de Groot and Brand (2001) to help force estimations on the shoulder in field condition in sports and industrial applications. More models are also being developed with application to a variety of sports (Graham-Smith & Lees, 2005).

Ergonomics principles were applied design evaluation of rowing machines to enhance safety during training (Bernstein et al, 2002). It was suggested that longer stroke lengths and greater forces are risk factors for soft tissue injuries. A detail discussion on science and football made by Reilly (2003) indicated significant development in the notational analysis of actions during football (soccer and other forms) matches. More suitable training designs were evolved in which the demands of the game and the fitness profiles of soccer players are placed in perspective (Reilly, 2005).

One of the most investigated area in sport ergonomics is racket sports since it has made unique challenge to scientists and have provided vehicles for developing scientific methodology (Lees, 2003). These research works had provided valuable inputs to implement training programmes to improve players' fitness; guide players in psychological preparation for play; inform players of the strategy and tactics used by themselves and their opponents; provide insight into the technical performance of skills; understand the effect of equipment on play; and accelerate the recovery from racket-arm injuries. Analysis of techniques was critically discussed by Lees (2002) in an earlier work.

Risk management is common ergonomics practice under industrial set up. However, the same principles could be of importance in preventing injury occurrences among amateur sports participants (Fuller & Drawer, 2004; Micheli et al, 2005). Heat stress is a real danger for sports persons especially in long distance running and cycling, and sports participation under hot-humid conditions. Design intervention was attempted to develop lightweight cooling vests (Webster et al, 2005).

It is clearly evident that sports ergonomics had made considerable progress in terms of knowledge base and many applications of the knowledge have also occurred.

3.0 ERGONOMICS PROGRAMME IN SPORTS IN DIFFERENT COUNTRIES

Although "Sports Ergonomics" is not taught as a complete subject in graduate or postgraduate courses in any part of the world, many universities offer this subject as part of various courses. Some examples are given below:

Sports Ergonomics (code no. SPMX710) is being taught as a paper in Sports Medicine at University of OTAGO, New Zealand. The courses that include this subject are Masters in Health Science and PG Diploma in Sports Science. Emphasis is given on interaction between the sports person and their environment (its effect on injury mechanisms and injury prevention including interaction with other participants), the surface on which the sport is performed, and equipment used.

A large number of Bachelor and Master courses are being conducted in UK through different universities. Details of these courses are available at International Sports Engineering Association website. The courses are mainly BEng or MEng in Sports Engineering. Bachelor and Master of Science courses in Sports Technology is also available.

In India no organization conducts a specialized course in Sports Ergonomics or Sports Engineering/Technology.

4.0 FUNDING POSSIBILITIES IN SPORTS ERGONOMICS

In the last few decades sports has invaded human life in a big way all over the world. It is estimated that the size of the sports industry in United States is $200 Billion and sports goods consist of $25.62 Billion (Business Today, 2005). According to the estimates the Indian Sports industry will become a Rs.40,000

Crore business by the year 2010. Of this amount spending on coaching is the highest followed by broadcasting rights and endorsement (BT, 2005). Unfortunately no estimate is ever given for the spending on scientific aspects of sports and that make a cause for deep concern.

5.0 FUTURE SCOPE AND CHALLENGES

Talk of ergonomics in sport would be futile unless it can generate awareness of the role of science in sports and commercial significance of academic pursuit of sports science. Sports events are watched by a major potion of the world population. Ergonomics application in sports can lead to awareness about "Ergonomics" among common public. This would lead to faster recognition of the subject in the country. It is obvious that such an effort would need success stories in Indian sports ergonomics. A few hurdles are to be crossed to get the precious success stories.

- Govt. support for Research and development in this field is most important step at present. It is a serious question that in the absence of even a national vision for "Ergonomics" how a part of the discipline can get support? Participation of industries in research and development would make a difference.

- Next question is "Where from the trained manpower will come? Fortunately first ever only "Ergonomics" programme has started in India (NITIE course). Majority of persons who has worked in this field came from Calcutta University, Dept of Physiology. They are basically physiologists with specialization in Work Physiology and Ergonomics. Two more Universities have started teaching ergonomics as specialization, Vidyasagar Uiversity and Kalyani Uiversity. Many engineering colleges have included Ergonomics as a part of their curriculum. In all these universities and colleges the focus is Industry or agriculture and not sports. It is required to start structured professional courses on "Ergonomics" to harness the strength of this specialized field for the enhancement of Indian sports performance.

- Academic or professional courses alone can not produce the technical manpower with advanced knowledge because of many limitations. Students need proper placement to practice the knowledge gain in an university and to convert the knowledge into technology or applications. Unless many research laboratories are established with advanced facilities comparable to other leading countries (in ergonomics) this would not be achieved.

- The incubation period for development of technology, based on research work, is big at present. It is the job of the ergonomists to reduce this period reasonably by designing efficient systems of to enhance the growth. One example may be considered. Match analysis was conceived in and around 1980. Selling of computerized equipment was started during the end of 90's. A period of 15-20 yrs was consumed to produce a marketable technology. Of course technology was less advanced when the concept started, but the later part of the growth was also not comparable with the speed of growth in technology.

- Application of ergonomics in sports would not happen without the support of Coaches, sports administrators and sports federations. Educating these people would create conducive environment for the growth of this specialized area of knowledge.

- Entrepreneurship programmes in Ergonomics is another way to generate many small units of ergonomics practitioners. Certification program in ergonomics is an undeniable requirement towards this path.

Development of knowledge is important, not how it is developed. Both 'sports medicine' and 'ergonomics' has helped in improving the sports performance in elite level as well as in leisure activities. Indian contribution to the knowledge on sports ergonomics is insignificant, but some attempts were made.

Acknowledgement

This article would not have been written unless urged by Dr. W. Selvamurthy, CC, DRDO, New Delhi. The support from Dr. P.K. Nag, NIOH, Ahmedabad and Prof. Nachiketa Sadhu, IDC, IIT, Mumbai, is memorable.

Bibliography

1. 2nd International Conference on Sport, Leisure and Ergonomics. 9-11 July 1991. Proceedings. Ergonomics. 1994 Jan; 37(1):1-229

2. A nations progress: Engineering to Sport. Business Today, Oct. 9, 2005, pp110-121.

3. Ahuja, A. and Goswami, A. Injury Index : an indicator of epidemiology in sports trauma. NIS Scientific Journal, 1993, 16, 4, 3, 8.

4. Alexander MJ, Boreskie SL. An analysis of fitness and time-motion characteristics of handball. Am J Sports Med. 1989 Jan-Feb; 17(1):76-82.

5. Annett, J., The learning of motor skills: sports science and ergonomics perspectives. Ergonomics, 1994, 37(1):5-16.

6. Atha J, Yeadon MR, Sandover J, Parsons KC. The damaging punch. Br Med J (Clin Res Ed). 1985 Dec 21-28; 291(6511):1756-7.

7. Frederick, E. C. Physiological and ergonomics factors in running shoe design Applied Ergonomics 1984, 15, 4, *281-287*.

8. Atha J. Current techniques for measuring motion. Appl Ergo. 1984 Dec; 15(4):245-57.

9. Bernstein IA, Webber O, Woledge R. An ergonomic comparison of rowing machine designs: possible implications for safety. Br J Sports Med. 2002 Apr;36(2):108-12.

10. Catalano, J.F., and Hanccock, P.A. The human factors of sport — a review. In: Proceedings of the Human Factors Society 27th Annual Meeting, Norfolk,

Virginia, 10–14 October 1983, edited by A.T. Pope and L.D. Haugh. The Human Factors Society, Santa Monica, California, 1983, pp 379–382.

11. Charteris, J., Candler, P. D. and Li, J-C. The V-scope ultrasonic motion monitor: ergonomics applications in occupational manual materials handling and clinical exercise therapy. *Applied Ergonomics 1994, 25, 1, 35-40.*

12. Clarys JP, Cabri J, de Witte B, Toussaint H, de Groot G, Huying P, Hollander P. Electromyography applied to sport ergonomics. Ergonomics 1988, Nov; 31(11):1605-20.

13. Cooke, Alison J. The Aerodynamics and Mechanics of Shuttlecocks. Ph.D. dissertation, University of Cambridge, UK, 1992.

14. Corlett, E.N. and Stapleton, C. (1999), The Ergonomics Society: 50 years of growth. Paper presented at the 1999 Ergonomics Society Annual Conference. Also published in Ergonomics, (2001), Vol. 44, No. 14, 1265-1277.

15. Davids, K., Smith, L. and Martin, R. Controlling system uncertainty in sport and work *Applied Ergonomics 1991, 22, 5, 312-315.*

16. de Groot JH, Brand R. A three-dimensional regression model of the shoulder rhythm. Clin Biomech (Bristol, Avon). 2001 Nov;16(9):735-43.

17. de Vey Mestdagh K. Personal perspective: in search of an optimum cycling posture. Applied Ergonomics 1998, Oct;29(5):325-34.

18. Goswami, A. Sports Ergonomics : Its nature and scope. UDYOG PRAGATI – The Journal for Practicing Managers 2001, 25, 2, 32-36.

19. Goswami, A., Ghosh, A.K., Ahuja, A. and Mathur, D.N., Movement and posture analysis in competitive sports. Proc. International Symposium on Ergonomics, Occupational Health, Safety and Environment, IIT, Bombay, Jan. 2 6,1991.

20. Graham-Smith P, Lees A. A three-dimensional kinematic analysis of the long jump take-off. J Sports Sci. 2005 Sep;23(9):891-903.

21. Hong Y, Robinson PD, Chan WK, Clark CR, Choi T. Notational analysis on game strategy used by the world's top male squash players in international competition. Aust J Sci Med Sport 1996, 28(1):18-23.

22. Hughes M, Franks IM. Dynamic patterns of movement of squash players of different standards in winning and losing rallies. Ergonomics 1994, 37(1):23-9.

23. Forkink, A. and Frings-Dresen, M. H. W. Measurement of oxygen consumption with the Cosmed K2: a comparative study *Applied Ergonomics1994, 25, 2, 95-100.*

24. Hughes, M.. Computerized notation analysis in field games. Ergonomics 1988, 31, 1582-1592.

25. Lees A. Technique analysis in sports: a critical review. J Sports Sci. 2002, Oct; 20(10):813-28.

26. Lees, A. Computers in sport. Applied Ergonomics 1985, 16, 1, *3-10.*

27. Micheli LJ, Glassman R, Klein M. The prevention of sports injuries in children. Clin Sports Med. 2000, 19(4):821-34.

28. Murrell, K.F.H. "Ergonomics: Fitting the Job to the Worker",1960.

29. Nigg, B.M., and Segesser, B. The influence of playing surfaces on the load on the locomotor system and on football and tennis injuries. *Sports Medicine*, 1988, **5**.6, 375–385

30. O'Donoghue, P. and Ingram, B. A notational analysis of elite tennis strategy. J. Sports Sci. 2001, 19(2), 107-115.

31. Page KA, Steele JR. Breast motion and sports brassiere design. Implications for future research. Sports Med. 1999, 27(4):205-11.

32. Reilly T, Gilbourne D. Science and football: a review of applied research in the football codes. J Sports Sci. 2003, 21(9):693-705.

33. Reilly T. Ergonomic aspects of sport and recreation. Can J Appl Sport Sci. 1981, 6(1):1-10.

34. Reilly, T. and Greeves, J. Sport, leisure and ergonomics: the Olympic cycle. Ergonomics 2000, 43(10), 1447-8.

35. Reilly, T. and Lees, A. Exercise and sports equipment: Some ergonomics aspects Applied Ergonomics 1984, 15, 4, 259-279.

36. Reilly, T. and Thomas, V. A motion analysis of work rate in differential roles in professional football match play. J. Human Mov't. Stud. 1976, 2, 87-97.

37. Reilly, T. Assessment of some aspects of physical fitness Applied Ergonomics 1991, 22, 5, 291-294

38. Reilly, T. Ergonomics in sport: An overview. Applied Ergonomics 1984, 15, 4, *243-244.*

39. Reilly, T. Sport, leisure and ergonomics : Burton, Cheshire, UK, 26–27 November 1987 • CONFERENCE *Applied Ergonomics 1988, 19, 2, 168.*

40. Thapliwal, V. Development of suitable methodology to evaluate skill and match play in hockey by using time motion analysis and physiological variables. Master of Sports Coaching Desertation, Punjabi University, 1991.

41. Reilly, T. Ergonomics and sport. *Applied Ergonomics 1991, 22, 5, 290.*

42. Sakurai, S. and Ohtsuki, T. , Muscle activity and accuracy of performance of the smash stroke in badminton with reference to skill practice. J. Sports Sci. 2000, 18(11), 901-914.

43. Shackel, B. Ergonomics from past to future: An overview. Proceedings of the Annual Ergonomics Society. Contemporary Ergonomics 1989, Presentation notes.

44. Shephard RJ. Sport, leisure and well-being—an ergonomics perspective. Ergonomics 1988, 31(11):1501-17.

45. Shephard, R.J. Fitness and Health in Industry. Karger, Basel, (Medicine and Sports Science, 21, Series Editors: M. Hebbelinck and R.J. Shephard) 1986a.

46. Shephard, R.J. . Economic benefits of enhanced fitness. (Human Kinetics Publishers, Inc., Champaign, Illinois)1986b.

47. Stuart J, Atha J. Postural consistency in skilled archers. J Sports Sci. 1990, 8(3):223-34

48. URL: http://ergonomics.org.uk

49. URL: http://www.ergoboy.com

50. URL: http://www.hfes.org/

51. URL: http://www.iea.cc/

52. URL: http://www.sportsengineering.org/

53. Webster J, Holland EJ, Sleivert G, Laing RM, Niven BE. A light-weight cooling vest enhances performance of athletes in the heat. Ergonomics. 2005, 10;48(7):821-37.

54. Yeadon MR, Atha J, Hales FD. The simulation of aerial movement—IV. A computer simulation model. J Biomech. 1990, 23(1):85-9.

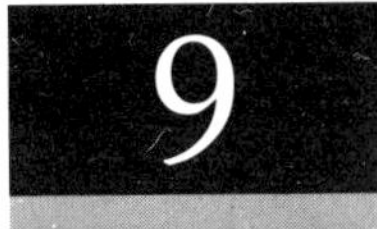

Sports Sciences: Irrefutable Realities of Modern Sport

M.L. Kamlesh

Retd. Principal
Laxmibai National Institute of Physical Education, Trivandrum

ABSTRACT

With its competitive aspect getting increasingly more intense, modern sport has become a warlike phenomenon with excellence or success its prime objective at all levels of participation.

The sport academics – coaches and trainers – have somehow come to get convinced that this warlike situation can't be handled deftly without the application of principles of such scientific disciplines as sports physiology, biomechanics, sport and exercise and psychology, nutrition, sports medicine and the like. Sport sans science is almost a non-entity. Identifying talent, developing and exploiting human potential for competitive sport, is virtually impossible without the athletes and trainers turning scientific in body, mind and behaviour. This calls for a complete rejuvenation of the teaching and training methodologies in exercise, active recreation and sports.

As an integrated activity of body and mind, sport is dealt with a host of sport sciences, some of which target general health and wellbeing of the people in general, while others focus on performance-enhancement in competitive sport. It has now been established beyond a shadow of doubt that competitive sport is the sole purview of a few *genetically endowed* individuals. On the basis of their value to the training of elite athletes, sport sciences are, by and large, categorized in (a) **critical sport sciences** such as biomechanics, physiology and psychology, and (b) **supportive sport sciences** like nutrition, sports medicine, anthropometry etc., each one having a specific place in the sport-science hierarchy.

Human beings are no run-of-the mill product; they are thinking and feeling biological machines that interact in an environment and to treat them as sporting robots will tantamount to putting cart before the horse. Consequently, it would be necessary to evaluate the ongoing athletic practices on the touchstone of scientific realities of sport and take cognizance of pros and cons of the induction of science in

> training of athletes in sports and at different levels of performance, without closing eyes on the human limitations and environmental constraints.
>
> The irreversibly changing sport scenario brings into focus the role of sport scientists in not only bringing to light, through constant research effort, the bright and gray areas of sport science knowledge – both general and specific – but also in *educating* the athletes and their trainers, and helping them build their training and competitive policies, practices and programmes on the realities of science. It would need them to create an atmosphere in which athletes and coaches and science faculty get increasingly closer and benefit from each other's experience. The test of their wisdom lies in knowing sport as much as they know science.

When an archer is shooting for enjoyment, he has all his skill; when he shoots for a brass buckle, he gets nervous; when he shoots for a prize of gold, he begins to see two targets.

Chuan Tzu – a Chinese sage.

SPORT AND SCIENCE

Like monozygotic siblings, sport and war have both dazed and fazed man for millennia, though for different reasons. No effort, how so powerful, has been able to eliminate war from man's existence; rather its reflections are unwittingly seen in sport. The unbridled instinct of pugnacity inherent in man often has made the most pleasant activity like sport fall on the borderline of war, and overshadowed its implicit motive of individual excellence and social enjoyment with an ever-increasing greed for winning in athletic contests as a mark of personal victory and national prestige. With its spontaneity and geniality vanishing for the reasons beyond comprehension and rational explanation, modern sport is hardly anything but "a sublimation of aggressiveness", and "the violence of cultured man" (Cohen, 1975). Cutthroat competition, in this tough Age, calls for tough approach in training and preparation for tough athletic exploits; it toughens athletes to make tough-climb to pinnacle of glory, a reality.

Beginning with the modern Olympics-1896 at Athens, the athletic records today seem to have *less* meaning than they had a few decades ago. Where as in the past a record may have stood for years, they are now being tumbled and re-written at an amazing speed. This dramatic change in athletic performance is generally attributed to the ever-ascendant use of science and technology in every important compartment of sport – from identification of athletic talent at a tender age, to grooming young athletes into star performers for a considerably long period, and to exposing them to progressively hard competitive situations in well-defined phases. At each of these watersheds, athletes are subjected to rigorous training which *inter alia* underscores innovative skill-acquisition, refined performance techniques, improved nutrition, high-class sports-medicine backup (especially in the realm of injury prevention and treatment), maintaining optimal energy thresholds (through consistent physiological conditioning and hard weight-training), perfecting mental skills, etc.

Highly impressed by and obsequiously true to the Greek ideals of aesthetics, ethics and athleticism, the founder of the modern Olympic Games – Baron Pierre de Coubertin – was actually wary of using science to "build athletes" (Schrof et al, 1996). He wanted athletes to use no *crutches* and compete in natural styles, and in the finest tradition of the ancient "Pan-Hellenic festivals" (Kamlesh, 2002). With fast-changing values of life, values in sport too have always been undergoing irreversible transformation over time. The Olympic Movement could not resist for long (1) approaching *induction of science* in training for competitive sport, and (2) dilution of amateurism by allowing inclusion of *professional* sports in the programme of events, with far reaching consequences for the world of sport at large.

Overshadowing the age-old *trial-and-error* technique based on rational thought process, the **Age of Scientific Approach** to athletic training began in the early forties of the twentieth century with a big bang. This made the sport academia and athletic fraternity go *performance-crazy*. As a result they started to conceive of and put into practice innovative techniques of preparing athletes for competitive endeavours by applying principles of science, mainly physiology to begin with, to enhance human movement potential. By 60's, the world of sport saw a host of sport sciences suddenly appearing on the scene and nowhere and empowering athletes from several East European countries (especially those from erstwhile Soviet Union, German Democratic Republic, Czechoslovakia, Poland etc.) to spring surprises in track & field, gymnastics, weight-lifting, swimming and other events at the Olympic Games, with "extensive as well as intensive sport science back-up" (Kamlesh, 2002). With an astute single-minded focus on athletic excellence, the shrewd sports academics, joined hands with the experts in biomechanics, anthropometrics, physiology, psychology etc., and began to re-align their line of thinking and recast their training methodologies with an aim to systematically identify, exploit, and manipulate every single variable that could ensure success at athletic competition. With these realties pervading the sport arena, the standard-bearers of the Olympic Movement ultimately gave in under the amounting pressure from all around. As a result, the International Olympic Committee had to recognize the importance of developing sport sciences. Going a step forward, it instituted awards and scholarships, which gave impetus to research on various aspects sport. The *Sport Administration Manual* of the IOC (1999, p. 385) reads thus:

As technology, medicine and science increasingly turn their attention to sport and high performance athletes, there are enormous quantities of new information available for the preparation of athletes for competition. These fields are becoming so complex, specialist scientists and physicians are working with those teams that have resources to spend these areas.

The unprecedented knowledge boom that followed development Kament of science and technology, in general, and their induction in physical activity and sport has greatly encouraged man push the boundaries of athletic performance beyond the "bounds of utmost human thought", with tremendous success, stunning the world on the one hand, and making sport all-science on the other.

Science is defined as nothing but "an organized and systematic accumulation of observation" (Sprinthall et al, 1991) or an "ordered knowledge of natural phenomena ..." (Damper, 1961) and the study of the relationships that exist between them. As in most fields of life, so in sport, no important aspect – infrastructure, equipment, sport-ware, sport-wear, management, training, organization and competition – has escaped the watchful eye of science. Wittingly or unwittingly, it is natural for some people to assume that 'the real competitors in sport are now not the athletes and their trainers but the engineers, physicians, equipment manufacturers' etc., (Perey, 1991).

The more the curve of sporting excellence moves up, the more the society's *lust for more* gets stronger, enjoining upon the athletes and their trainers to take recourse to innovative techniques that facilitate manufacture and use of more modern equipment, employment of harder training regimes, and better biotechnologies to give their ability and skill to perform a cutting edge, though sometimes at the cost of some other risk to life.

For the scions of sport, the ***best test for sport*** is to:

- strive for the ultimate human performance;
- use modern technology to aid performance;
- strive for better times;
- attempt to break records;
- aim for optimum health among athletes;
- promote faster recovery from injuries; and
- make performance more efficient.

To be able to stand the stringent tests of time in terms of efficacy and efficiency, there is no way out for the votaries of sport excellence but to use crutches of the sciences such as biomechanics, sport and exercise physiology, sport psychology, and others for the steep climb. The rise of various offshoots of sport sciences is, perhaps, the most dazzling reality of modern sport.

Sport Sciences

Sport sciences are no foreign intrusion, nor are they superficialities of academic exercise. They are research-oriented data-based innovative strategies proposed and employed by *clear, clever and creative* minds towards integrating science with sport in such a manner that the athletes and their trainers are facilitated in potentiating their effort to the unknown limits in their effort to achieve excellence at various stages of athletic competition. Over the decades, sport sciences have multiplied in number, each one evolving into a highly specialized as well as applied area of knowledge. Sometimes termed as *hybrid* sciences because of their intermediacy or buffer-like situation between two different disciplines, they are remarkably devoted to 'identifying, understanding, investigating, analyzing, and applying relevant facts of science in an effort to bring about performance-enhancement in physical activity, exercise and sport at different levels and various stages'. They are developing "training technologies to give athletes *competitive edge*", as Perey (1991) put it. Under the ideal conditions, they offer expert scientific backup for top sport training and performers. Perey (1991) and Schrof et al (1996) believe that with ever-increasing scientific inputs:

> *Scientists hope to use technology to tailor perfect techniques for each athlete. Computer simulations may allow them to invent new devices or swimming strokes and discover changes as revolutionary as the Folsbury Flop that could completely alter the way that sport is performed today.*

Society has come to view human body as an *invincible machine*. Physiologically, the human body is not designed as a machine, and therefore should not be expected to perform the way a machine does. A machine can repeat a movement several thousand times without the risk of breakdown but the human body can't. When scientists use quantities in function, such as joint angles and pressure points, to design equipment that will perform the best mechanically, human factors can be overlooked. This machinelike view of the body poses the problem that humans, unlike machines, have tendons, cartilage, muscle, fat, a limited energy supply, anxiety and human emotion, all of which affect performance of the skill (Rintala, 1995). Athletic performance, therefore, is no simple question of learning, practicing and mechanically performing physical skills; it has physiological, psychological, and socio-cultural aspects also, which can't be kept aside while developing specific performance techniques.

The modern athletes – whether professional or amateur, mediocre or elite – swim and *run faster, throw farther* and *jump higher*, as the Olympic motto reads; and they do so more efficiently economizing on their energy, than their predecessors could. These improvements, feels Michael Meyees of the West Texas A & M University, USA, are attributed to several inter-related factors such as:

- smarter nutrition,
- a greater understanding of biomechanics of sport movement,
- better training techniques,
- advances in psychological support, and
- improvement in coaching education.

Continuing efforts to extend laboratory research into sport-specific field setting have resulted in identification of several variables deemed necessary for successful performance in several sports (Coyle, 1995; Foreman, 1989; Mahood et al, 2001; Schabort et al, 2000). The adoption of this message of **science and sweat** has been slow for a variety of reasons:

1. Sports performance testing is expensive.
2. Facilities are limited to the elite class of athletes, generally out of general public reach, and every day coach's budget.

3. The opportunity to combine cutting-edge sport science technology with the traditional field and court assessment has never been easier, and is much more readily accessible to today's progressive thinking coach.

EXERCISE SCIENCE AND/OR SPORT SCIENCE

In the hierarchy of sciences, there is no sport science category but any branch of science, in some way connected with and harnessed to making human movement more efficient, economical and precise, may legitimately qualify to find in the galaxy of sport sciences, so to say. From the experience of the sports academia, it is now well understood that some branches of science have a much warmer relationship with exercise and sport performance than others. Consequently, application of scientific principles is considered by examining at least four branches of sciences – biomechanics, physiology, psychology and interdisciplinary approaches – although this knowledge is applied differently to each of the exercise and sport disciplines.

Exercise Science

The concept of Exercise Science emerges from the application of the principles of science to understanding and analyzing human movement in terms of its energy cost and making movement efficient and economical as part of the physical activity programmes aiming to ensure well-being of the people.

Exercise Science is the study of human movement as related to exercise, (recreational) sport and physical activity. It is dedicated to promoting and integrating scientific research and education on the health benefits of exercise; and, its delivery of physical activity programmes that prevent disease, facilitate rehabilitation, promote health, and enhance human capability for performance. Exercise Science is a part of the field of Sports Medicine, which also includes clinical areas of study. Important contributions made by exercise scientists to sports medicine include:

- Muscle-fibre typing (so crucial for deciding aerobic or anaerobic workouts for an individual).
- Testing of maximal aerobic capacity and cardiac output.
- Studies of blood flow, lactic acid metabolism and temperature regulation.
- Analysis of muscle fatigue.
- Research on muscle hypertrophy, and bone density.
- Measurement of body composition.

One of the major focuses of Exercise Science is the study of responses and adaptations that occur with exercise. The exercise scientist or physiologist can predict how fast the heart will beat with various types of exercises. He is able to explain many of the chemical and physical changes that cause the increased heart rate.

Sport Science

The more critical application of scientific knowledge is reflected in *Sport Science*, which offers scientific support for top sport training and performers in all sports. The difference between exercise science and sport science is not *generic* but qualitative. The canvas of sport sciences is appreciably quite broad, and many more fields of knowledge are trying to find some slot there. However, disciplines like physiology, nutrition, psychology, medicine etc. – to count a few – have evolved well. They develop training technologies that intend to enhance performance and give athletes the *competitive edge* (Perey, 1991). The training methods devised under the sport science head help to prevent injury and reduce the recovery time between workouts. Special machines, for instance, can be used during training to precisely control the velocity of an athlete's movement to prevent damage to the joints. '**Less pain and more gain**' is now the emphasis of training for athletes, with greater importance being placed on training efficiency' (Sheppart, 1988).

The distinction between exercise science and sport science is just skin- deep, rather translucent, for a scientist in any field of knowledge can address to issues of exercise and competitive sport in equal measure and with the same dexterity. Therefore, categorizing exercise scientists and sport scientists into distinctly separate is simply preposterous and, perhaps, meaningless. A qualified sport and exercise scientist can expect to have a broad technical, physiological and psychological knowledge, and he stands to benefit from current developments within the field offering a professional status that is recognized world wide.

The phenomenal rise of sports medicine and sport science as emerging potential areas of study and research during the last fifty years augurs well with what future holds for the sport and exercise scientists in the 21st century.

Marked *individualized* exercise prescription for the prevention of diseases, and ensuring sound health and well being for all, shall become order of the day.

- Courses in exercise, nutrition counseling will assume an increasingly important role in medical school curricula and in the training of physicians.
- Exercise, sport and sport science curricula at institutes of physical education and sports shall attune itself to the emerging facts about human motion and create tremendous pressure for course-diversification.

DICHOTOMY OF SPORT SCIENCES

Considering excellence as the major objective of competitive sport, it is well-recognized that the magnitude of potential changes in athletes diminishes as performance standards increase and that any improvement in performance at elitist level of sport, if at all, will not occur without a strong support from physiology, biomechanics, and psychology, which in Rushall's view (1989) are **critical enhancement sports sciences**. Rushall also refers to sciences like medicine, anthropometrics, nutrition, biochemistry etc., as **supportive** ones for their role in solving several problems of the athletes. Yet he cautions:

> *In practical situations it is difficult to determine whether performance improvements occur because of changed fitness levels (a physiological contribution), altered skill enactments (better biomechanical features), or improved behavioral/appraisal factors (a psychological contribution).*

Traditionally, Rushall (1989) to argue that there has been a form of **"pecking order"** for sport sciences and their importance for training athletes. Physiology is emphasized in most courses of study more than other two enhancement sciences. It is easily measured, has response forms that are consistent across individuals, and produces easily recognized response characteristics in athletes. For example, if an athlete sweats then a coach knows that he/she is doing something to the athlete. With the advent of slow-motion video the analysis of skill has been improved. Coaches now can quickly recognize changes in style or technique properties from trial to trial. As skills are developed (taught) the bio-mechanist can claim influence on those changes. Such direct attributions are used to substantiate the value of those sciences for performance changes in athletes. Sport psychology is an emerging enhancement science and must be emphasized when maximum performances are desired. The greater the muscle-mind coordination, the more qualitative the performance output, is a psychological truism. *Athlete development systems and programmes are no longer adequate if they only emphasize skill and physical development.* The inclusion of sound psychological principles and practices in training and competition preparations and conduct is a necessary ingredient of modern sport.

Relative Contribution of Critical Sport Sciences to Athletic Success

In order of their ascending criticality to success in sport, enhancement sciences may be listed thus – biomechanics, physiology and psychology.

Biomechanics

Biomechanics is a diverse interdisciplinary field, with branches in Zoology, Botany, Physical Anthropology, Orthopedics, Bioengineering and Human Performance. The general role of biomechanics is to understand the mechanical cause-effect relationships that determine the motions of living organisms. In relation to sport, biomechanics contributes to the description, explanation, and prediction of the mechanical aspects of human exercise, sport and play. Over the years, it has assumed the stature of a sport science, which applies the laws of physics and mechanics to human performance, in order to gain greater understanding of team as well as individual sports events through modelling, simulation and measurement. This science has expanded rapidly over the past twenty-five years, with its roots traced to various established disciplines such as engineering, anatomy, aerospace, rehabilitation, medicine, orthopedics, sport science and many others.

A typical biomechanics laboratory hosts a broad array of research foci that encompass several sub-domains of the discipline. The major thrusts include the application of biomechanical principles to motor control and neurological problems, understanding how muscle properties dictate the coordination of movement, exploring the mechanical behavior of musculoskeletal structures at the tissue level, and exploring innovative solutions to orthopaedic problems.

In sport scenario, biomechanics is all about developing organic power; mechanics of skill performance, and refining play dynamics involving power, rhythm, speed, timing etc. Record-breaking performances especially in individual sports such as swimming, athletics, gymnastics etc., are attributed to a greater use of principles of biomechanics in acquiring and performing perfect stroke mechanics.

Neither physical educators nor sports coaches can do without banking upon biomechanics in teaching mechanically perfect skills and developing training techniques for athletes. By and large, the application of the principles of biomechanics enables physical educators and athletic trainers to:

    (a) *chart out* interrelations between form and function of the body while developing motor skills and athletic skills in young athletes, and make them perform them more precisely and efficiently;

    (b) *planning skill-teaching* in consideration of the relationship between body mechanics and kinesiology and other basic sciences; for instance, physiology and bio-chemistry; and

    (c) *investigating and understanding human movement* by means of concepts of classical physics and their derivatives in the practical arts of engineering, in order to improve physique and movement skills.

One area of major concentration over the past few years has been the biomechanical analysis where coaches and athletes have traditionally used video cameras and videocassette recorders to scrutinize and improve their performance. Today computers and high-tech devices are available to retrieve, analyze, replay, edit and print the desired performance into three dimensional (3D) stick figure images that are analyzed from different angles without the need for VCR. In almost all sporting events movements can be digitally assessed in the indoor, outdoor or under-water environment. Opportunities for several kinds of performance assessment exist with the help of a personal computer.

> *The key, however, is the ability to merge both experience of the coach with the objectivity of the analyzed sport movement to create a plan for athletic performance enhancement.* **But 'returns from biomechanics diminish, if no innovative skills are introduced. With time, the ability to improve through mechanical efficiency lessens'** *(Rushall, 1986).*

Exercise/Sport Physiology

Sport physiology is often referred to as *Exercise Science*. It applies physiological concepts basically connected with exercise dynamics to an athlete's training and performance. At very best, it studies how the body's structures and functions are altered when exposed to acute and chronic bouts of exercise. While ***acute responses*** to training involve how the body responds to one bout of exercise, ***chronic physiological adaptations*** to training mark how the body responds over time to the stress repeated exercise bouts.

Key points: Acute Responses to Exercise:

- Control environmental factors such as temperature, humidity, light, and noise;
- Account for diurnal cycles, menstrual cycles, and sleep patterns;
- Use of ergo meters to measure physical work in a standardized condition;
- Match the mode of testing to the type of activity the subject normally performs.

Exercise and sport physiology develops the energy basis for performance but is limited and does not change its potential for effect after a relatively short period of time (Astrand & Rodahl, 1977). One of its major focuses is the study of responses and adaptations that occur with exercise. The exercise physiologist can predict how fast the heart will beat with various types of exercises and he can also explain many of the chemical and physical changes that cause the increased heart rate.

Its contribution to performance enhancement is unbelievably unique because of the fact that exercise performance testing is marked by utmost objectivity, precision and clarity. To be competitive, the key is to select tests (or monitor those physiological variables) that, when conducted under natural or simulated laboratory conditions, provide information to the particular sport, position or event (Muller et al, 2000).

From the viewpoint of physiology, the ***Basic Training Principles*** involve:

- *Individuality*: Consider the specific needs and abilities of the individual (sportsperson).
- *Specificity:* Training adaptations are highly specific to the type of activity and the volume and intensity of training.
- *Disuse*: Include a programme to maintain fitness.
- *Progressive overload*: Increase the training stimulus as the body adapts.
- *Hard/easy:* Alternate high-intensity with low-intensity workouts.
- *Periodization:* Cycle specificity, intensity and volume of training.

The most important services that are readily attracting coaches' attention these days are the evaluation of pulmonary function, nutritional analysis, electro-cardio-graphic workup, and total blood chemistry. The use of treadmill for assessment of cardio-respiratory parameters has made sport performance testing an easy and every day affair.

A few *important contributions made by Exercise Scientists* to sports medicine include:

- Muscle-fibre typing (so crucial for deciding aerobic and anaerobic workouts for an athlete with event-specificity)
- Testing of maximal aerobic capacity and cardiac output
- Studies of blood flow, lactic acid metabolism and temperature regulation
- Analysis of muscle fatigue
- Range of motion (ROM) testing
- Research muscle hypertrophy, and bone density
- Measurement of body composition

Irrefutable databased evidence as to the efficacy of exercise and sport physiology has largely come both from longitudinal, and cross-sectional studies (the former being more accurate) as well as from laboratory research and field research.

By defining physiological parameters, it is possible to make some predictions regarding performance capabilities, assess an athlete's predisposition to injury, critically review the effect of current training protocols, and provide the coach with additional insight and a competitive edge over those programs relying primarily on subjective criteria' (Roetert et al, 1995.

Sport Psychology

Sport psychology *involves the connection between the mind and the body and the utilization of this connection for enhancing athletic performance. Emphasis is placed on the understanding of the psychological and physiological parameters, which the athlete can utilize to enhance his or her performance skills.* These days it is now a *buzzword* in sport. It is a field of knowledge that enables athletes to **dream** (dream realistically about performing in their sport beyond their known capacity), **believe** (what would seem possible under the existing set of circumstances). In its broadest sense, sport and exercise psychology 'determines how well the finite contributions of physiology and biomechanics are used. It is the critical sport science for governing the level of performance that will occur' (Rushall, 1989).

A right mindset is one of the determinants of an athlete's performance - right along with his or her physical condition and technical skills. *Just as there is a set of well-known physical characteristics of a champion* (i.e. strength, speed, stamina), *there is a set of mental factors identified as part of a winner's mindset.* They are confidence, concentration, consistency and control. Mindset is very important for several reasons:

- It is often this factor that sets apart the best from the good.
- Research has revealed that at least 50 percent of the athletic performance successes and even more athletic performance errors and failures are due to mental factors.

- Often times talents plus physical and technical training can take athletes and teams only so far before they reach a performance plateau. It is mental training that will carry them to the next level.

With time sport psychology seems to be moving away from the narrow mental forces to a study of the links between the body and the mind. ***It is becoming more motoric than psychological.*** It is developing techniques and tactics that may help, for example, tennis players to hit the ball where they want, how they want and when they want. More precisely, it defines ideal performance state, and helps the athletes to build it up and maintain it. It can help trigger the correct response via visualization and imagery rituals.

One of the focuses for future sport psychology will be an increasing use of athletic personality profiling (Vanden, 1993; LeUnes, 2000). Athletes involved at all levels of sport, experience all kinds of stresses, distractions, high levels of expectations and physical challenges etc. Various psychometric instruments such as Profile of Mood States (POMS), Athletic Coping Skills Inventory (ACSI), Sports Inventory for Pain (SIP) etc., have been utilized by an increasing number of sport scientists, medical personnel, and coaches to assess coping skills, motivation, self-esteem, pre-competition anxiety, and mood relevant to sport.

The relative merit of the ***supportive sport sciences*** such as nutrition, health sciences, sports medicine, sport sociology, and others can't be underplayed both in academic interactions and competition training.

Laboratory Testing in Sport Sciences

For athletic trainers, supplementing standard field and weight-room testing as well as athletes' individual experiences with what is derived from the sport science laboratory is an important consideration. This may enable them substantiate their own personal observation on athlete's potential and the extent to which it can be further developed with inputs from different sport sciences. No one on earth should underestimate the trainer's insight, understanding and judgment. Assessing them for validity, on the anvil of the objective scientific observation (testing, measurement and evaluation), has an important place in the scheme of things in sport. However, in order to utilize effectively the available sport science support the athletic trainers need to keep a number of things in mind.

1. Communicate with the sport science personnel as often as possible and select testing variables that are relevant to your sport. Neither ape others, nor keep your eyes off your objectives. The mode of testing, the rate of motion, the physical resistance selected, the specific muscles used, and the range of motion experienced by the athlete should closely resemble the actual sport.

2. Let tests be challenging, but not to the point where test termination results in excessive body temperature, dehydration or fuel depletion or even mental exhaustion.

3. Select testing techniques that are valid and reliable especially in case of psychological variables, rather than based simply on familiarity and tradition.

4. Insure that the tests are conducted in a safe and productive atmosphere to optimize player safety, concentration and instruction.

5. Both the sport scientist and the sports academic must ensure that proper feedback, in adequate measure, is provided to the athlete in time by those he/she trusts.

6. Respecting human rights of all athletes is important; no testing should trespass ethical limits.

There is no perfect test nor can testing be perfect. There will always be limitations in predicting athlete's performance. Although an athlete may give 100% during laboratory testing, there is no substitute for the actual competitive environment. Further, the information derived from the sport science laboratory should be an adjunct and, if performed accurately, should be an important piece of decision-making process in evaluating an athlete. Test should never stand alone when dealing with the complex environment of sport competition.

References

Astrand, P.O. & Rodahl, K. (1977) *Textbook of work physiology*. New York: McGraw Hill.

1. Cohan, John (1975) Psychological aspects of sports with particular reference to variation in performance. In H.T.A Whiting (Ed.) *Readings in Sports Psychology*. Lepus Books.

2. Coyle, E.F. (1995) Integration of the physiological factors determining endurance performance ability. *Exercise and Sport Science Reviews*. 23: 25-64.

3. Damper, W.C. (1961) *A history of science and its relation with philosophy and religion*. (4th Ed.) Cambridge, England: Cambridge University Press.

4. Foreman, K. (1989) The use of talent-prediction factors in the selection of track and field athletes. In Gambele V. (Ed.) *The Athletic Congress's Track and Field Manual*. 31-36, Champaign, Il; Leisure Press.

5. Kamlesh, M.L. (2002) *Foundations of physical education*. New Delhi: Metropolitan.

6. LeUnes, A. & Burger, J. (2000) Profile of mood states research in sport and exercise psychology: past, present and future. *Journal of Applied Sport Psychology*. 12: 5-15.

7. Mahood, N.V. et al (2001) Physiological determinants of cross country racing performance. *Medicine and Science in Sports and Exercise*. 33(8); 1379-1384.

8. Meyes, Michael West Texas. A & M University, U.S.A.

9. Muller, E. et al (2000) Specific fitness training and testing in competitive sports. *Medicine and Science in Sports and Exercise*. 32(1): 216-220.

10. Perey, T. (1991) Bio-mechanically engineered athletes. *Spectrum*. 27: 43-44.

11. Pretoire South African Association for Sports, Physical Education and Recreation.

12. Rintalla, J. (1995) Sport and technology: Human questions in a world of machines. *Journal of Sport and Social Issues.* 19:1, 62-75.

13. Roetert, E.P. et al (1995) Establishing percentiles for junior tennis players based on physical fitness testing results. *Clinics in Sports Medicine.* 14(11): 1-21.

14. Rushall, Brent S. (1986) Program consideration for training superior athletes. In *proceedings of the International symposium of research in sport and recreation.*

15. Rushall, Brent, S. (1989) Sport psychology: The key to sporting excellence. *International Journal of Sport Psychology.* 20: 169-190.

16. Schabort, E.J. et al (2000) Prediction of triathlon race time from laboratory testing in national triathletes. *Medicine Science in Sports and Exercise.* 32(4): 844-849.

17. Schrof, J.M. et al (1996) *The winning edge.* U.S. News & World Sport. 121: 3 8 - 49.

18. Shapport (1988) *Sport Quest.*

19. Sprinthall, Richard C. et al (1991) *Understanding educational research.* Englewood Cliffs, New Jersy.

20. Vandan, Auweele Y. et al (1993) Elite performers and personality: from description and prediction to diagnosis and intervention. In Singer, R.N.; Murphy, M; Tennet, C.K. (Eds.) *Handbook of research in sport psychology.* 252-289. New York: MacMillan.

10

Comparison of a Linear and a Daily Undulating Periodized Training Program for Maximal Strength in Male Air Force Cadets

Petros Bilios[1], Dimitrios Soulas[2], Kiriakos Taxildaris[3], Vassilis Gerodimos[2] and Gregory C. Bogdanis[4,5]

[1]Hellenic Air Force Academy; [2]Department of Physical Education and Sports Sciences, University of Thessaly; [3]Department of Physical Education and Sports Sciences, University of Thrace; [4]Department of Sports Medicine and Biology of Physical Activity, University of Athens; [5]Ergometry Laboratory, Hellenic Air Force Academy, Hellas

ABSTRACT

The purpose of present study was to compare a Linear (LP) and a Daily Undulating Periodized (DUP) strength training program aiming to increase maximal strength. Forty five healthy male cadets of the Hellenic Air Force Academy (aged 18-22 y) were randomly assigned to a LP group (n = 15, height: 176.3 ± 6.8 cm, body mass: 77.0 ± 9.6 kgr; mean ± SD), a DUP group (n = 15, 176.2 ± 5.0 cm, 77.2 ± 7.3 kgr) or a control (C) group (n = 15, 176.5 ± 8.5 cm, 75.5 ± 9.0 kgr). One repetition maximum (1RM) bench press strength and body composition were measured before and after 8 weeks of bench press training that involved four sets three times per week. Every two weeks, the LP group gradually decreased the repetitions (from 10 to 4) and increased resistance (from 70% to 90% of 1RM), while the DUP group followed the same pattern, but also altered the repetitions (2 -15) and load of training (60-95% of 1RM) on a daily basis. The weekly volume and intensity were equated for each training program. Data were analyzed using a two Way analysis of variance with repeated measures. Body fat and body mass were similarly decreased in all groups (p < 0.01), but fat free mass remained unchanged. A significant but similar improvement in 1 RM bench press strength was observed in the two experimental groups but not in C (LP: 8.1 ± 1.2%, DUP: 10.8 ± 1.7%, C: 2.3 ± 2.1%). This data suggest LP and DUP strength training is equally effective in increasing maximal bench press strength in healthy young males.

INTRODUCTION

Weight training is one of the most appealing and effective forms of exercise for the improvement of muscle strength in many sports (Fleck et al., 1997) and is commonly used to increase fitness for performance of military duties (Kraemer et al., 1995 & Schiotz et al., 1998). Although the most effective training scheme for developing muscular strength has not been precisely determined, most strength and conditioning professionals agree that strength training programs should be periodized (Willoughby, 1993 and Plisk & Stone, 2003). Periodization is a method of manipulating intensity and volume of training in different periods or cycles within a complete training program (Baechle & Earle, 2000). There are various types of periodized programs due to the numerous possible configurations of the program variables, e.g. the combination of the number of sets and repetitions the exercises performed, or the training frequency. Currently, Linear Periodization (LP) and Daily Undulating Periodization (DUP) are two of the most commonly used types of periodization (Rhea et al., 2002). Briefly, LP involves increasing training intensity gradually, while training volume is decreased within and between cycles. DUP is characterized by changes of intensity and volume on a weekly or daily basis (Baechle & Earle, 2000).

Only a few studies have directly compared the effects of LP and DUP with conflicting evidence. Some of these studies found no difference in strength increases between LP and UP programs (Baker et al. 1994 & Hoffman et al. 2003), while others demonstrated superiority of the DUP program (Rhea et al., 2002 and Kraemer et al., 2000). The purpose of present study was to compare a LP and a DUP strength training program aiming to increase maximal strength in a relatively short period of time (8 wk). To isolate the effect of periodization from the influence of parameters such as exercise specificity and total training load, only one exercise was trained and tested, while training intensity and volume were equated in the two periodized programs.

METHODOLOGY

Participants

Forty five healthy male cadets of the Hellenic Air Force Academy aged 18-22 y, with at least 6 months of weight training experience volunteered for this study, which had ethical approval. After signing an informed consent form, participants were randomly assigned to a LP group (n = 15, height: 176.3 ± 6.8 cm, body mass: 77.0 ± 9.6 kg; mean ± SD), a DUP group (n = 15, 176.2 ± 5.0 cm, 77.2 ± 7.3 kg) or a control (C) group (n = 15, 176.5 ± 8.5 cm, 75.5 ± 9.0 kgr).

Preliminary Measurements

One repetition maximum (1RM) bench press strength and body composition were measured before and after training. A period of one week was utilized for familiarization and preliminary testing. Body mass was measured to the nearest 0.1 kg on a medical scale (Seca 770) with subjects in shorts. Skinfold thickness was measured at seven sites (chest, midaxillary, triceps, subscupular, abdominal, anterior suprailiac and thigh) using a John Bull caliper and body composition (fat and fat-free mass; FFM) was then estimated (Jackson & Pollock, 1978, Siri, 1956).

A one Repetition maximum (1 RM) bench press test was conducted. [As described by Beachle and Earle (2000)]. Subjects warmed up with a light resistance, then achieved a 1 RM effort within 3-5 attempts. No bouncing of the bar on the chest was permitted. Bench press testing was performed on a standard supine free-weight bench press station. The subject lowered an Olympic weightlifting bar to midchest, then pressed the weight until elbows were fully extended. Previous studies have demonstrated good test-retest reliabilities ($rs > 0.90$, Hoffman et al., 1990, 1991). No 1 RM determinations were made for the complementary exercises. No injures were observed in any test. The same investigators performed all pre- and post-training tests at the same time of the day.

TRAINING PROTOCOL

Training was performed 3 days per week for 8 weeks (24 sessions) according to a Linear Periodization and a Daily Undulating Periodization method. Every two weeks, the LP group gradually decreased the repetitions (from 10 to 4) and increased resistance (from 70% to 90% of 1RM), while the DUP group followed the same pattern, but also altered the repetitions (2 -15) and load of training (60-95% of 1RM) on a daily basis.

The LP group performed 4 sets of (70% 1RMx10 rep) during weeks 1-2, 4 sets of (80% 1RMx8 rep) during weeks 3-4, 4 sets of (85% 1RMx6 rep) during weeks 5-6 and 4 sets of (90% 1RMx4 rep) during weeks 7-8. The DUP group altered training on daily basis (Monday: 4 sets of 80% 1RMx 6rep; Wednesday: 4 sets of 60%1RMx15rep; Friday: 4 sets of 70%1RMx 10rep during weeks 1-2. Accordingly, the program for the next weeks for the DUP group was as follows (Monday, Wednesday, Friday): 4 sets of 85%1RMx6rep; 4 sets of 65%1RMx12rep and 4 sets of 75%1RMx8rep during weeks 3-4; 4 sets of 90%1RMx4rep; 4 sets 70%1RMx10rep; 3 sets of 80%1RMx6rep during weeks 5-6; 4 sets of 95%x2rep; 3 sets of 75%1RMx8rep; 4 sets of 85%1RMx4rep during weeks 7-8. The C group followed the normal physical activity program of the Air Force Academy that involved general physical conditioning with no specific strength training elements during that period.

Each session of the two training groups included one core (bench press) and 3 other exercises for the muscle groups of the upper body. In these various assistance exercises only 12-15RM loads were used. Workouts consisted of one warm-up set followed by 3-4 sets for each of the four exercises with 1-3 min of rest between sets. There were no differences between experimental groups in the total volume or relative intensity either for core or assistance exercise. The training frequency and session duration were standardized during the experimental period. After 4 weeks a new 1 RM test was performed and the individual training load was adjusted accordingly. All training sessions were supervised by one of the investigators. None of the subjects suffered any injuries during the study. Compliance to the training program was 100% for all groups.

STATISTICAL ANALYSES

Statistical analyses of the data were accomplished utilizing two-way analyses of variance (group x time) with repeated measures on one factor (time: pre and post training). Tukey's post-hoc tests were performed where appropriate to locate pairwise differences. Significance level was set at $p < 0.05$.

RESULTS

Body fat and body mass were similarly decreased in all groups ($p < 0.01$), but fat free mass (FFM) remained unchanged (Table 1).

Table 1 Pre and post training measurements of body mass, body fat and fat free mass for the two training groups (LP, DUP) and the control (C) group. * $p < 0.01$ from PRE

	Body mass (kg)		Body fat (%)		Fat free mass (kg)	
	Pre	Post	Pre	Post	Pre	Post
LP	77.0±2.5	76.1±2.1*	16.7±1.0	15.7±0.8*	64.0±1.8	64.0±1.7
DUP	77.2±1.9	76.0±1.8*	14.8±0.8	13.7±0.7*	65.7±1.3	65.4±1.1
C	75.5±2.3	74.1±2.2*	14.2±0.8	13.6±0.7*	64.7±1.8	64.0±1.9

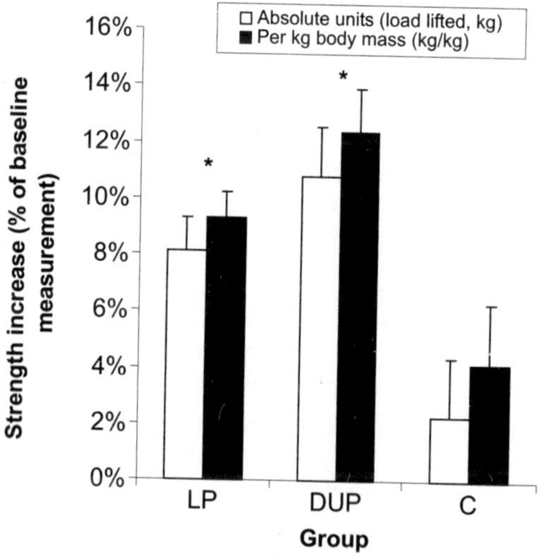

Fig. 1 Percent improvement relative to the baseline measurement (PRE) either expressed in absolute units (load lifted in kg) or in relative units (load lifted per kg body mass) for the two training groups (LP and DUP) and the control group (C). * $p < 0.01$ from LP and DUP.

One RM bench press strength per kg body mass (BM) was 1.02 ± 0.04 kg/kg BM, 0.99 ± 0.05 kg/kg BM and 1.13 ± 0.08 kg/kg BM, for the LP, DUP and C group, respectively. A significant but similar improvement in 1 RM bench press strength was observed in the two experimental groups but not in C (Fig. 1). This improvement was similar when expressing strength as absolute units (kg lifted) or relative units (per kg of body mass or fat free mass).

DISCUSSION

The pre- to post-training FFM response in the current study are similar to the results reported by Rhea et al (2002) who reported no significant difference in FFM for pre to post following the 12-week RT program in both DUP and LP. With the exception of one study (Baker et al. 1994), most other studies reported no significant difference in FFM for individuals following DUP or LP programs for a similar length of time. This is probably a function of training volume that was higher in that study. The significant increase in strength without an increase in FFM would indicate neural adaptations supporting the idea that significant increases in strength can occur without muscle hypertrophy in the early stages of a RT program (Behm, 1995; Burger & Burger, 2002 and Chestnut & Docherty, 1999).

The present study showed that both DUP and LP training programs are effective methods for increasing 1 RM strength, without any significant difference between the two programs. These results agree with findings of previous studies (Baker et al. 1994 & Hoffman et al. 2003) that reported no significant difference in strength gains between LP and undulating periodized (DUP). Although there was a tendency in the DUP group for a higher increase in strength (Fig. 1), this was not statistically significant. It is likely that the differences between the LP and DUP training programs were not severe enough to elicit statistically significant differences. Peterson et al. (2006) reported the DUP to be significantly superior to the LP ($p < 0.05$) in increasing strength in trained males. This may suggest that this type of periodization may provide marginally better results, but further research is needed to support this argument.

In summary, this study has shown that both LP and DUP training programs result in a similar increase in maximal bench press strength in 24 training sessions, without any increase in FFM. The tendency for a greater effectiveness of DUP warrantees further investigation.

Reference

1. Baechle, T. B., and Earle, R. E. (2000). Essentials of strength training and conditioning. (2 Ed). Champaigh. IL. *Human Kinetics.*

2. Baker, D., Wilson, G., and Carlyon, R. (1994). Periodization: the Effect on Strength of Manipulating Volume and Intensity. *Journal of Strength and Conditioning Research,* 8, 235-242.

3. Behm, G.D.(1995) Neuromuscular implications and applications of resistance training. *Journal of Strength and Conditioning Research*, 9, 264.

4. Burger, A.M., & Burger, M.S. (2002). Neuromuscular and hormonal adaptations to resistance Training: Implication for strength development in females athletes. *National strength & Conditioning Association*, 24, 51-59.

5. Chestnut, J. L.,& Doherty,D. (1999). The effects of 4 and 10 repetition maximum weight-training protocols on neuromuscular adaptations in untrained men. *National Strength & Conditioning Research*, 13, 353-359.

6. Fleck, S. J., and Kraemer, W. J. (1997). Designing resistance training programs, 2nd Ed. Champaign, IL., *Humans Kinetics*.

7. Hoffman, J.R., Wendell M., Cooper J., and Kang J. (2003). Comparison Between Linear and Nonlinear In-Season Training Programs in Freshman Football Players. *Journal of Strength and Conditioning Research*, 17(3), 561-565.

8. Jackson, A.S., and Pollock, M.L. (1978). Generalized equations for body density of men. *British Journal of Nutrition*, 40:497-504.

9. Kraemer W. J., Ratamess, N., Fry, A. C., McBride, T. T., Koziris, L.P., Bauer, J. A., Lynch, J. M.,Fleck , S. J.(2000). Influence of Resistance Training Volume and Periodization on Physiological and Performance Adaptations in Collegiate Women Tennis Players, *The American Journal of Sports Medicine*, Vol. 28, No 5, 626-633.

10. Kraemer, W. J., Patton, J. F., Gordon, S. E., Harman, E. A., Deschenes, M. R., Reynolds, K., Newton, R. U., Triplett, N. T., Dziados, J. D. (1995). Compatibility of high-intensity strength and endurance training on hormonal and skeletal muscle adaptations. *Journal of Applied Physiology*, 78:976-989.

11. Peterson, M., Rhea, M., Alvar, B., Dodd, D. (2006). Undulation training for development of hierarchical fitness and improved job-specific testing performace: a firefighter readiness initiative and recommendation. In proceedings of 5th International Conference on strength training. Aagaard, P., Madsen, K., Magnusson, P., Bojsen- Moller, J(Ed). *Strength Training for Sport, Health, Aging and Rehabilitation*, pp. 241-242. University of Southern Denmark.

12. Plisk, S.S., & Stone, M.H. (2003). Periodization srategies. *Strength and Conditioning Journal*, 25, 19-37.

13. Rhea, R. M., Ball, D. S., Phillips T. W., Burkett, N. L.(2002). A Comparison of Linear and Daily Undulating Periodized Programs with Equated Volume and Intensity for Strength, *Journal of Strength and Conditioning Research*, 16(2), 250-255.

14. Schiotz, M. K., Potteiger, J. A., Huntsinger, P. G., and Denmark, Lt, C. D. C.(1998). The short-term effects of periodized and constant-intensity training on body composition, strength and performance. *Journal of Strength and Conditioning Research*, 12(3), 173-178.

15. Siri WE (1956) The gross composition of the body. In C.A. Tobias & J.H. Lawrence (Eds.), Advances in biological and medical physics (vol. 4, pp. 239-280). New York: Academic.

16. Willoughby, D.S. (1993), The effects of Mesocycle-Length Weight Training Programs Involving Periodization and Partially Equated Volume on Upper and Lower Body Strength. *Journal of Strength and Conditioning Research*, 7(1), 2-8.

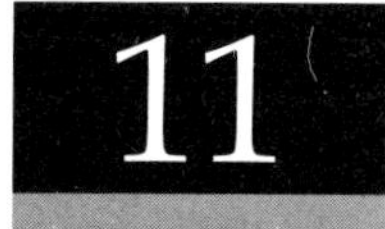

Endurance and Strength Training during the Pre-Season Period in Greek Professional Soccer Teams

G. Pidoulas, D. Soulas, K. Taxildaris, A. Kampas and V. Voutselas

Department of Physical Education and Sports Science, University of Thessaly, Karies, Trikala 42100, Greece.

ABSTRACT

Soccer is one of the most widely played sports in the world and the players need a combination of technical, tactical and physical skills to succeed. The pre-season preparation period in soccer lasts from five to eight weeks and it differs from country in country. The aim of the present research was to record the training methods used by Greek professional soccer teams to improve endurance and strength performance.

Data was collected from the 16 professional soccer teams of the Greek Super League. Data collection was performed by interview, including closed type questions. One way ANOVA was used to examine the differences in training sessions.

The eight weeks of physical preparation in Greek elite soccer showed that the most frequent type of endurance training without ball weeks was long slow distance training performed. After the third week the most frequent type of training is the intermittent training ($p < 0.05$). Moreover, the most frequent type of endurance training with ball is intermittent training ($p < 0.05$). As far as strength training is concerned circuit training seems to be the most prominent type of training for the first week of the preparation period, whereas after the third week the most frequent type of training is training for muscle hypertrophy and power performed ($p < 0.05$).

Traditionally during pre-season build-up, aerobic endurance seems to be regarded as the foundation on which fitness is built, with interval training following up as the most commonly used method to develop aerobic endurance. Endurance training for soccer players carried out using small-sided games in an intermittent form might additionally develop technical and tactical skills similar to situations experienced during the game and was expected to show a greater volume of training. Two different mechanisms, muscular hypertrophy and neural adaptations are central in the development of muscular strength in soccer. As neural adaptations show greater impact on rate of force development and performance in terms of accelerations the time used for hypertrophy training might be questioned.

INTRODUCTION

Soccer is one of the most widely played sports in the world and players need a combination of technical, tactical and physical skills to succeed (Hoff, Helgerud, 2004). However, studies that have been undertaken concerning soccer performance improvements, have often focused on technique and tactics at the expense of physical resources such as endurance, strength and speed (Helgerud, Engen, Wisloff, Hoff, 2001). The importance of aerobic ability in professional soccer is highlighted by the fact that elite players cover 10-12 km during a competitive match at an average intensity of around 75% of their maximal oxygen uptake (VO_{2max}). In addition, aerobic system contributes approximately 90% of the total energy cost of match play (Helgerud, et. al 2001).

The main aim for the trainer should be on the one hand the appropriate preparation of soccer players in order to be ready at the beginning of the competitive period and on the other hand to maintain a good fitness level during the championship period (Bangsbo, 1994).According to Bompa (1999) the period of preparation is divided in: a) general preparation (the general adaptation) b) special preparation (the special adaptation) based on the different characteristics of training. The aim of each period is different from each other as for the type and the intensity of training. This is the reason why the training program should be planned accordingly (Kraemer, Hakkinen, 2002).The pre-season preparation period in soccer lasts from five to eight weeks and is a different situation from country to country (Bangsbo, 1994). In the years to come soccer will most likely develop even further in a direction that demands more muscle strength and power (Andersen, 2006). During a game, professional soccer players perform about 50 turns, comprising forceful contraction, to maintain balance and control of the ball again defensive pressure (Withers, Maricic, Wasilewski et all, 1982). Hence, strength and power share importance with endurance at top level soccer play (Stolen, Chamari, Castagna, Wisloff, 2005). Power is in turn, heavily depended on maximal strength with an increase in the latter, being connected with an improvement in relative strength and therefore with improvement in power abilities (Buhrle, 1985).

In the modern bibliography everyone realise abundance of theories that is reported so much in the organisation of training process, but also methods of improvement of natural situation in the football. The aim of the present research was to record the training methods used by Greek professional soccer teams to improve endurance and strength performance.

METHODS

Data collected from the 16 professional soccer teams of the Greek Super League. Data collection followed the method of interview which included questions of closed type. In particular interviews collected information about the frequency of weekly training sessions for the improvement of physical condition with and with out ball as well as the methods that were employed and also, about the frequency of weekly training sessions for the improvement of strength as well as the methods that were employed.

One way ANOVA was used to examine the differences in training sessions between the eight weeks of physical preparation.

RESULTS

Data showed that the most frequent type of training ($p < .05$) without the use of a ball (Fig. 1), the first two weeks was long duration drills (3.69 ± 1.35 & 2.759 ± 1.0 sessions/day, for the 1st and 2nd week, respectively). After the third week, the most frequent type of training was the intermittent training (2.00 ± 0.97 sessions/day). Data are presented analytically in Table 1.

Moreover, the most frequent type of training ($p < .05$) with ball (Fig. 2) was the interval training (2.44 ± 1.03 & 2.38 ± 0.81 sessions/day, for the 3th and 4th week, respectively). Data are presented analytically in Table 1.

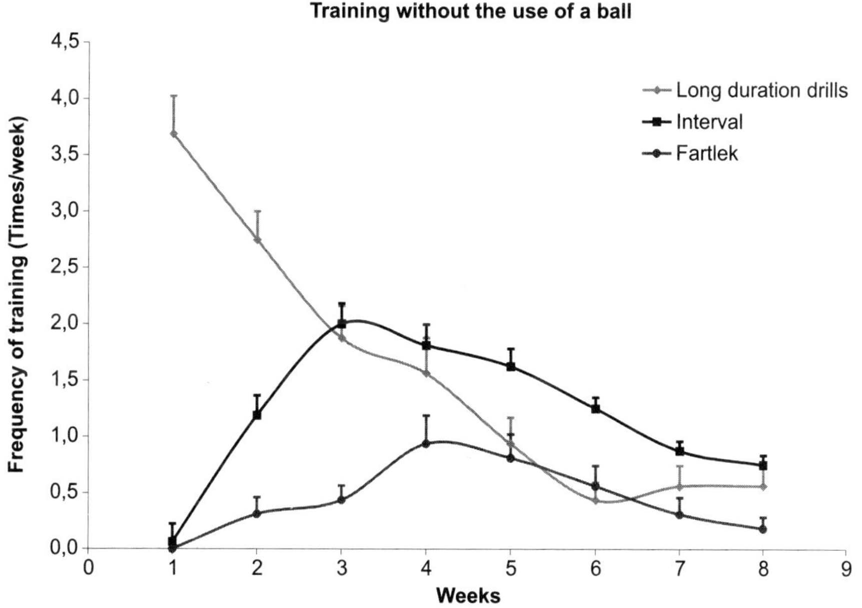

Fig. 1 Training methods without the use of a ball during the eight week physical training preparation period

Table 1 Training methods followed from 16 professional soccer teams during the eight week physical training preparation period. Data are presented as Mean±SD.

Weeks	Strength Training (training sessions/week)								Total (training sessions/ period)
	1	2	3	4	5	6	7	8	
Circuit Training	1.69±1.20	1.0±1.10	0.50±0:82	0.38±0.72	0.38±0.72	0.31±0.60	0.19±0.40	0.19±0.40	4.63
Muscle Hypertrophy	0.00±0.00	1.25±1.24	1.19±1.17	0.69±1.08	0.38±0.72	0.25±0.58	0.38±0.50	0.38±0.50	4.50
Muscle Coordination	0.00±0.00	0.00±0.00	0.13±0.34	0.63±0.81	0.75±0.86	0.56±0.73	0.06±0.25	0.38±0.50	2.19
Plyometrics	0.00±0.00	0.56±1.03	1.00±0.89	1.13±0.89	1.25±0.68	1.06±0.68	0.38±0.62	0.19±0.54	5.56
Power	0.13±0.52	0.00±0.00	0.73±0.70	1.33±0.62	1.27±0.59	1.07±0.46	0.40±0.51	0.53±0.52	5.47
Training without of the use of a ball (training sessions/week)									
Long Duration	3.69±1.35	2.75±1.00	1.88±1.15	1.56±1.26	0.94±0.93	0.44±0.63	0.56±0.73	0.50±0.63	12,38
Interval	0.07±0.26	1.19±1.11	2.00±0.97	1.81±0.98	1.63±0.81	1.25±0.86	0.88±0.72	0.75±0.58	9,57
Fartlek	0.00±0.00	0.31±0.60	0.44±0.51	0.94±1.00	0.81±0.83	0.56±0.73	0.31±0.60	0.19±0.40	3,56
Training with ball (training sessions/week)									
Long Duration	0.13±0.50	0.00±0.00	0.00±0.00	0.00±0.00	0.00±0.00	0.00±0.00	0.00±0.00	0.00±0.00	0,13
Interval	1.09±1.16	2.00±1.10	2.44±1.03	2.38±0.81	2.19±0.83	1.81±0.54	1.38±0.50	1.19±0.40	14,47
Fartlek	0.00±0.00	0.13±0.34	0.19±0.40	0.19±0.40	0.00±0.00	0.00±0.00	0.00±0.00	0.00±0.00	0,63

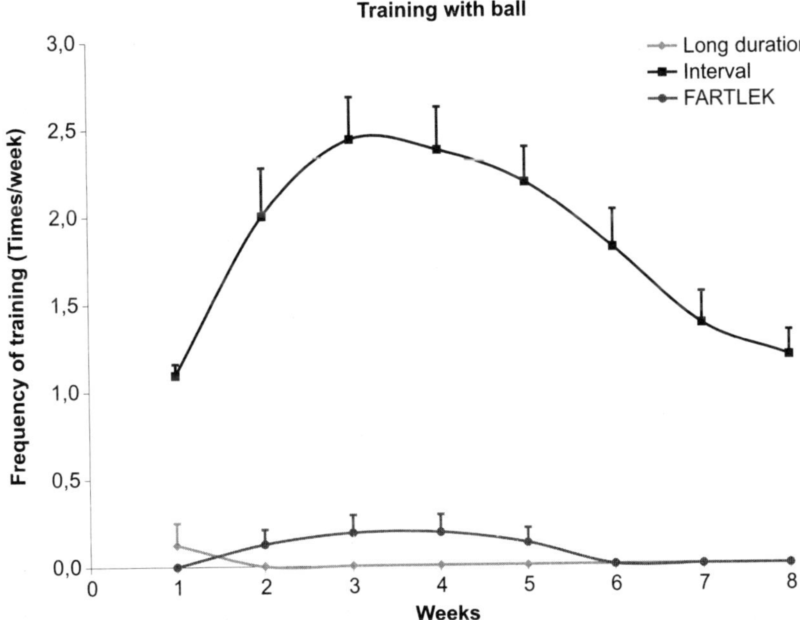

Fig. 2 Training methods with ball during the eight week physical training preparation period.

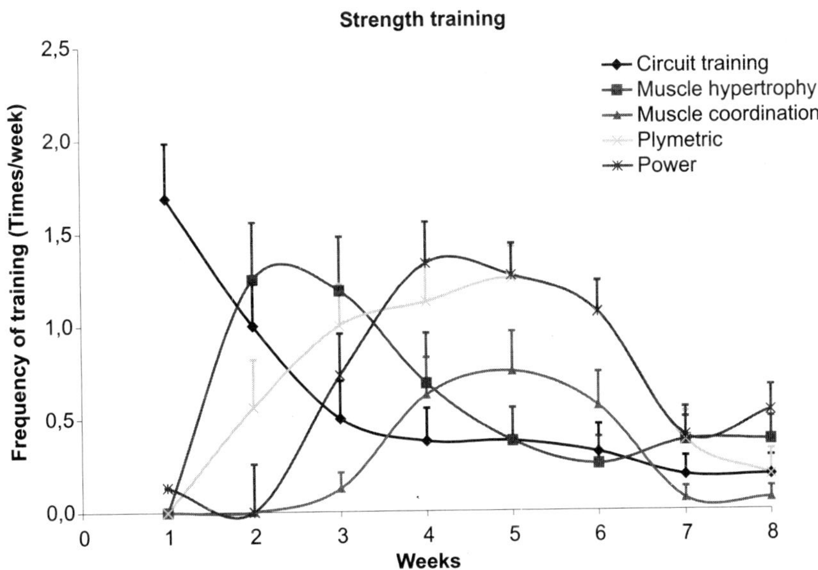

Fig. 3 Strength Training methods during the eight week physical training preparation period.

As far as strength training (Fig. 3) is concern circuit training seems to be the most prominent type of training for the first week of the preparation (1.69 ± 1.20 sessions/day) (p < .05). After the second week, the most frequent type of training was muscle hypertrophy (1.25 ± 1.24 sessions/day). Furthermore, after the forth week, the most frequent type of training (p < .05) was power (1.33 ± 0.62 sessions/day). Data are presented analytically in Table 1.

DISCUSSION

Physical conditioning is the process of developing physiological capabilities for a particular sport. Increasing a soccer player's fitness through training is a complex process that requires an increase in both aerobic and anaerobic energy capabilities (Dupont et al., 2004).

According to our result the most frequent type of training without the use of a ball the first two weeks was long duration drills. In the first 2-4 weeks of preparation the importance should be given in the improvement of basic endurance. This type of training should be placed in the beginning of preparation specifically in the first two, three weeks (Haffner 1990).After the third week of the pre-season build-up, aerobic endurance is regarded as the foundation on which fitness is built, with interval training being the most commonly used method to develop aerobic fitness (Coutts & Sirotic, 2004).

Nowadays in football training we use the interval method because the adaptations correspond with the conditions of a soccer game, and can be applied at the period of preparation in combination with the method of long duration for the improvement of basic endurance (Weineck, 1997).In the international bibliography we meet many protocols about interval training that are used for the improvement of endurance of the footballer (Helgerud et al, 2001., Hoff & Helgerud, 2004., Astrand et al 2003., Sassi, Reilly, Impellizzeri, 2003).

Specific soccer-related conditioning involves training players to deal with soccer situations on the basis of what is required in a given match situation (Verheijen, 1998). Training may range from technical/technical drills training through to small-sided games. Small-sided games or skill-based conditioning, especially during the pre-season, may provide a practical alternative to the current emphasis placed on traditional interval training for improving both aerobic and anaerobic fitness, (Coutts & Sirotic, 2004., Bangsbo, 2003., Reilly & Gilbourne, 2003., Helgerud, Engen, Wisloff, Hoff, 2001., Impellizzeri et al., 2006).

Several methods that improve strength training are used in the modern soccer. According to our results circuit training seems to be the most prominent type of training for the first week of the preparation. This method combines the simultaneous improvement of parameters of physical conditioning such as strength, speed, and endurance. After the second week, the most frequent type of training was muscle hypertrophy.

Power seems to be the most prominent type of training after the forth week. Power is the ability to produce as much force as possible in the shortest possible time and constitute for the footballer a very important factor of physical condition (Stolen et al., 2005). Power has big effect in the ability of acceleration and explosive strength and for the improvement we use the plyometric method (Buhrle, 1985).

The results of this study indicated the most frequent type of training and the methods that the team used in the pre-season period in Greek League. It is difficult to specialize which type of training we have to follow in the pre-season, because this must be judges by the coach and/or the individual of players.

References

Andersen, J. (2006). Planning of strength training in soccer players: Considerations and important aspects. 5th International conference on strength training. pp: 5-8.

Bangsbo, J. (1994). Endurance training in soccer: Periodisation in pre-season. pp: 283-290. Ho- Storm, Bagvaed

Bangsbo, J. (Reilly, T. and Williams, A. M. eds). (2003). Physiology of training. Science and soccer pp. 47-58. London

Bompa, T. (1999). Periodization. Theory and Methodology of training, pp: 193-202.Kendall /Hunt Publishing Company.

Buhrle, M. (1985). Grundlagen des Maximal – und Schnellkrafttrainings. Hofmann, Schorndorf.

Coutts, A., & Sirotic, A (2004). A comparison of a small games training versus interval training for improving aerobic fitness and prolonged, high intensity intermittent running performance. Paper presented at the Australian Association Exercise and Sport Science, Brisbane.

Dupont, G., Akakpo, K., & Berthoin, S. (2004). The effect of in-season, high-intensity interval training in soccer players. Journal of strength and conditioning Research, 18(3), 584-589.

Haffner, R., (1990): Fubball Ferienfreizeiten für jugendmann-schaften. Fubballtrainig 4, 54-59.

Helgerud, J. Engen, L.C. Wisloff, U. Hoff, J. (2001). Aerobic endurance training improves soccer performance. Medicine and Science in sport and exercise; 33: 1924-1931

Hoff, J., Helgerud, J. (2004). Endurance and strength training for soccer players. Sports Med; 34 (3): 165-180.

Impellizzeri, F., Marcora, S., Castagna, C., Reilly, T., Sassi, A., Iaia, F., and Rampirini, E. (2006). Physiological and performance effects of generic versus specific aerobic training in soccer players. Intemation of Sports Medicine 27, pp: 488-492.

Kraemer, W., Hakkinen, K.(2002). Strength training for sport: Periodization of training. pp: 69-91. Blackwell Scienc Ltd.

Reilly, T. and Gilbourne, D. (2003). Science and football: A review of applied research in the football codes. Sports Sciences 21, pp. 693-705.

Sassi, R., Reilly, T., & Impellizeri, F. (2003). A comparison of small-sided games and interval training in the elite professional soccer players. Communication to the Fifth World Congress of Science and Football, Lisbon, 11-15 April.

Stolen T, Chamari K, Castagna C, and Wisloff U. (2005). Physiology of soccer. Sports Med: 35 (6) 510-536 pp. 1.

Verheijen, R. (1998). Conditioning for soccer. Leeuwarden: Uitgeverij Eisma Bv.

Weineck, J. (1997). Training of football: Endurance training. pp: 95-111. Salto publishing company.

Withers, RT, Maricic Z, Wasilewski S, et al, (1982). Match analysis of Australian professional soccer players. J Hum Mov Stud; 8: 159-76.

12

A Study to Compare the Post Exercise Heart Rate Recovery between Coronary Artery Disease Risk Factors and Normal Adults

Ravinder Narwal, G.L. Khanna and R. Jeyasunder

Faridabad Institute of Technology

Manav Rachna Educational Institute, Faridabad

ABSTRACT

The present study was conducted to determine the effect of coronary artery disease risk factors on post exercise heart rate recovery in asymptomatic coronary artery disease risk factors young adults and making comparison with normal young adults.

Sixty subjects of age group 20-30 years were allocated into four groups (Normal, Overweight, Positive family history, and Hypertension groups) on the basis of Body Mass Index (BMI), Blood Pressure (BP), Family history. Each group consisted of 15 subjects. Heart Rate and blood pressure were measured before, during and after exercise up to 5 minutes of recovery periods.

Heart Rate Recovery (HRR) in normal group is fast as compare to Coronary Artery Disease (CAD) risk factors groups. Hypertensive group show slowest HRR between all the groups. Overall heart rate recovery mainly occurs in 1st minute and only the 1st minute of heart rate recovery can differentiate between normal and CAD risk factors groups. Results of heart rate recovery during 2nd,3rd, 4th and 5th minutes show no significant difference ($p > 0.05$) between normal and Coronary Artery Disease (CAD) risk factors groups

HRR after 85% Target Heart Rate (THR) can be used as a diagnostic, prognostic and therapeutic tool in young asymptomatic individuals.

INTRODUCTION

The incidence and prevalence of coronary artery disease are high enough to warrant consideration of a screening strategy, and the consequences of undetected disease are important.[1] At least 25% of coronary patients have sudden death or nonfatal myocardial infarction without prior symptoms. Therefore, the search for coronary patients who are asymptomatic, could potentially benefit from intensive primary prevention efforts is critically important.[2]

Heart Rate Recovery (HRR) is the declining of heart rate during the first five-minute following the completion of 85%THR (sub maximum exercise test). How quickly the heart rate recovers after treadmill exercise testing, remains a subject of much interest over the last few years for normal, CAD risk factors and sports persons.[6,7,8]

Heart rate recovery is mainly thought to be a function of vagal (i.e., parasympathetic nervous system) reactivation, with a delayed Heart Rate Recovery (HRR) reflecting a reduction in vagal tone.[8,9]

Limited information is available about the studies related with asymptomatic young age individuals having CAD risk factors and making comparison between normal subjects and CAD risk factors subjects based on HRR. Therefore, the purpose of this study is to compare the post exercise heart rate recovery between normal and asymptomatic coronary artery disease risk factors subjects.

This study is a part of cardiovascular disease prevention program and based on three time-honored classical coronary heart disease (CHD) risk factors: hypertension, overweight, and positive family history and approved by the research committee of Manav Rachna education institution.

METHODS

Asymptomatic subjects who had any one coronary artery disease risk factor (hypertension: Stage-1, overweight, positive family history) and normal subjects with age 20 to 30 years, Hemodynamicaly stable, without any pathology, able to comprehend and run on treadmill were included in this study. Subjects who had infections, musculoskeletal problems, Respiratory problems like Asthma; COPD, Cardiac arrhythmias, secondary hypertension, other coronary artery disease risk factors, any drug history, vestibular disorders i.e. vertigo, dizziness etc. were excluded from this study. Non-cooperative subjects were also excluded. All the subjects from Manav Rachna Educational Institute were evaluated and those met the inclusion and exclusion criteria and consented to participate in the study were included in the study. A convenient sample of 60 subjects were taken and assigned into four groups- Group A (CAD risk factors group) And Group B (normal group). CAD risk factors group was further divided into three subgroups i.e. overweight group, positive family history group and hypertensive group. Data was collected with Polar heart monitor and Sphygmomanometer (Diamond Deluxe 10-300 mm Hg).

PROCEDURE

The complete assessment of subjects was taken to rule out any contraindication or to detect any pathology before starting the test. Wet Chest strap transmitter was fixed on the subject's chest and receiver was tested for HR reading.

After demonstration, subjects were instructed to run on treadmill up to 85%THR according to Cleveland Clinic Choronotropic Assessment Exercise Protocol[27]without any chest symptom. The exercise test was terminated at a mandatory heart rate limit of 85% APMHR (age predicted maximum heart rate) or 9 on the 0-10 Borg scale, after which the exercise was discontinued.

Resting BP (by Standard Sphygmomanometer) and HR(by Polar Heart Monitor) measured after 5 minutes rest in supine position before exercise. During running on treadmill, BP and HR measured up to the completion of 85% Target Heart Rate. After this, subjects were allowed to lie down on the couch. The drop of heart rate and blood pressure were recorded during the first five minutes of post exercise recovery.

RESULTS

To investigate between-group differences, one-way analysis of variance (ANOVA) was used followed by Bonferroni post hoc comparisons where appropriate. Significant level was defined at (p<0.05) and the 95% confidence interval

1. HRR_1- Comparison of heart rate recovery in 1st minute during post exercise recovery period:

    Mean values and standard deviation for normal, overweight, positive family history, hypertension for HRR in 1st minute are 38.27 ± 9.17, 21.6 ± 4.95, 20.07 ± 5.12, 14.93 ± 4.31b/m respectively and f value for 1st minute recovery is 39.97. The observation of these values shows that there are highly significant differences among all the groups for heart rate recovery in 1st minute. (Fig. 1)

    Comparison of HRR between normal and CAD risk factors groups during 1st minute of recovery period. (Post hoc Bonferroni)

    Recovery of normal group in 1st minute is 18.2 beats > (more than) family history group, 23.3 beats > hypertension group, 16.6 beats > overweight group. This result shows that HRR is good in normal as compare to CAD risk factors groups.

    Within CAD risk factors groups, recovery during 1st minute shows that there is no significant difference between overweight and family history (p > 0.05), and between hypertension and family history (p > 0.05). Along with this, results also shows significant differences between overweight and hypertension groups i.e. (p < 0.05) and mean difference is 6.67 i.e. recovery in overweight is 6.67 beats more than hypertension group. (Fig. 2)

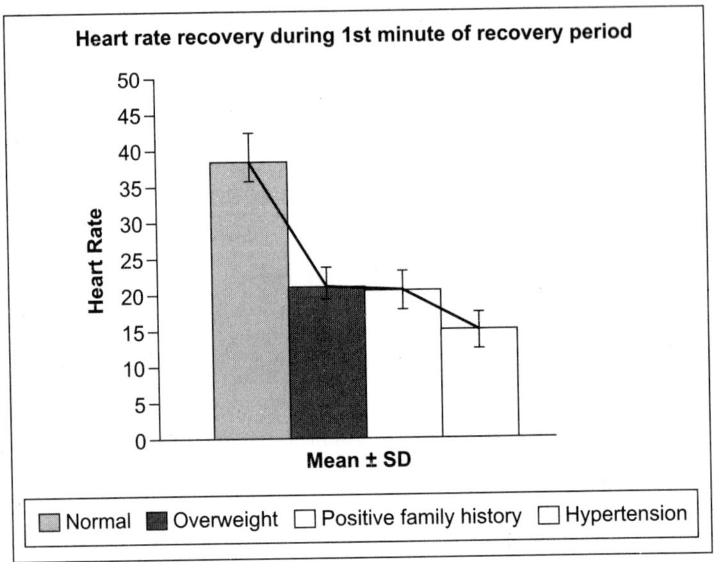

Fig. 1

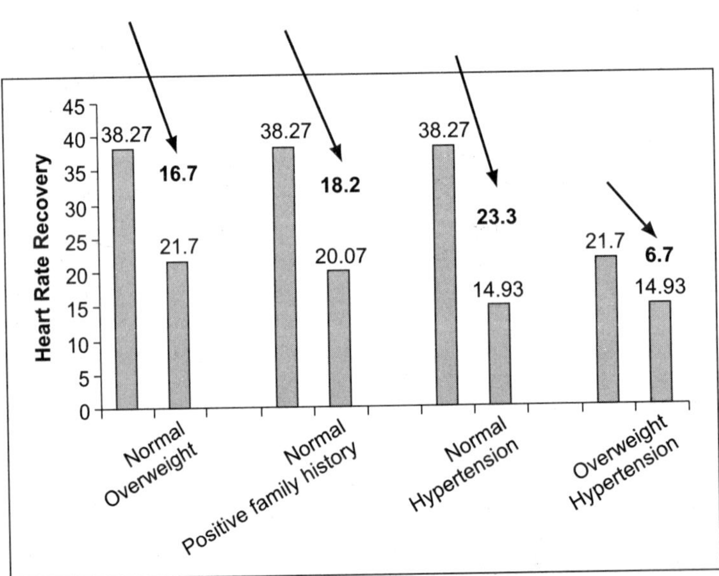

Fig. 2

2. HRR$_2$-Heart rate recovery in 1st two minutes during post exercise recovery period:

Mean values and SD for normal, overweight, positive family history, hypertension for heart rate recovery in 1st two minute are 54.13 ± 8.31, 36.47 ± 5.78, 38.13 ± 5.78, 29.07 ± 6.89 respectively and f value in 1st two minutes is 37.713. The observation of these values shows that there are highly significant differences between the groups for heart rate recovery in 1st two minutes. (Fig. 3)

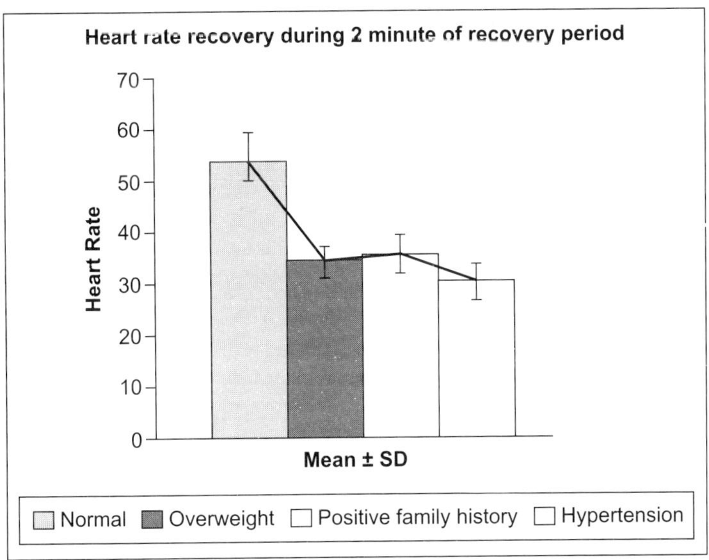

Fig. 3

3. HRR$_3$-Heart rate recovery in 1st three minutes during post exercise recovery period Mean values and standard deviation for normal, overweight, positive family history, hypertension for heart rate recovery in 1st three minute are 63.79 ± 8.5, 50 ± 7.56, 50.33 ± 7.39, 42.73 ± 7.88 respectively and f value in 1st three minutes is 18.037. The observation of these values shows that there are highly significant differences among all the groups for heart rate recovery in 1st three minutes. (Fig. 4)

4. HRR$_4$-Heart rate recovery in 1st four minutes during post exercise recovery period:

   Mean values and standard deviation for normal, overweight, positive family history, hypertension for heart rate recovery in 1st four minutes are 70.6 ± 9.77, 57.8 ± 6.88, 58.2 ± 9.18, 52.6 ± 7.48 respectively and f value in 1st four minutes is 12.37. The observation of these values shows that there are highly significant differences among all the groups for heart rate recovery in 1st four minutes. (Fig. 5)

5. HRR$_5$-Heart rate recovery in 1st five minutes during post exercise recovery period:

   Mean values and standard deviation for normal, overweight, positive family history, hypertension for heart rate recovery in 1st five minute

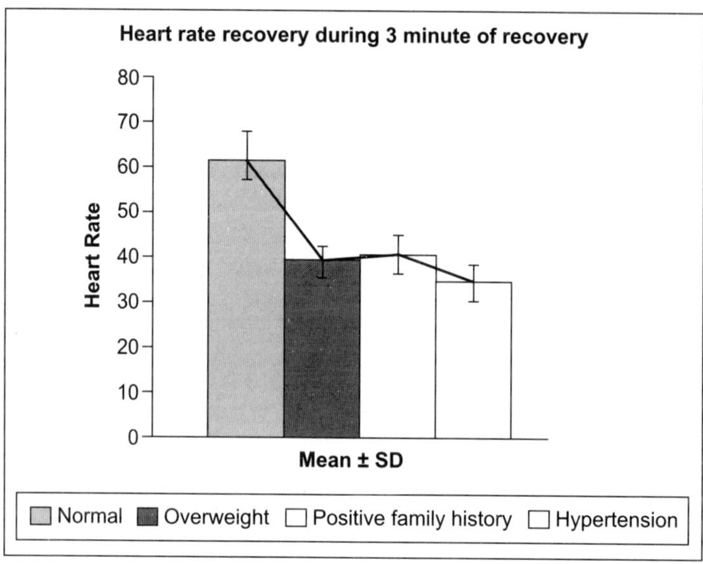

Fig. 4

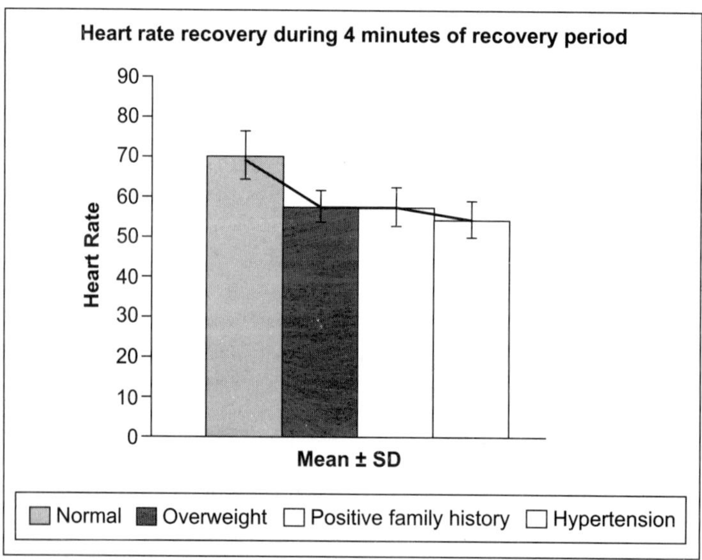

Fig. 5

are 75.93 ± 8.86, 65.0 ± 9.1, 65.2 ± 10.3, 59.87 ± 7.51 respectively and f value in 1st five minutes is 8.454. The observation of these values show that there are highly significant differences among all the groups for heart rate recovery in 1st five minutes (Fig. 6)

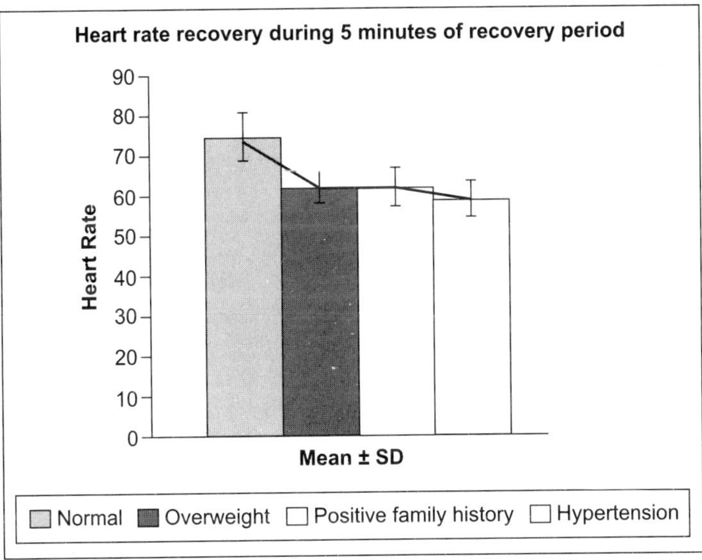

Fig. 6

6. Comparison of resting heart rate, 85% target heart rate achievement time, heart rate transient and peak exercise heart rate and heart rate recovery among all groups:

Comparison between mean data of resting heart rate, 85% target heart rate achievement time, heart rate transient and peak exercise heart rate show no significant differences (p > 0.05) among all groups. Mean data of heart rate recovery (from one to five minute) show highly significant differences (p < 0.05) among all groups. (Table 1, Fig. 7)

Results show that resting heart rate and heart rate change during exercise among all groups are same. Heart Rate Recovery (HRR) only the factor which differentiate normal group from Coronary Artery Disease (CAD) risk factor group that is, HRR in normal group is very

Table 1 Level of significance p < 0.05

Mean	Normal	Overweight	Positie family history	Hypertension	Pvalue
Target achievement time in minutes	7.6	6.5	6.3	6.8	0.141
Resting heart rate	76.2	76.8	78.2	74.6	0.15
Peak heart rate	163.	162.7	162.9	162.5	0.834
Heart rate recovery in one minutes	125	141	143	147	0.001
Heart rate recovery in two minutes	110	126	125	134	0.001
Heart rate recovery in three minutes	100	112	113	120	0.001
Heart rate recovery in four minutes	93	104	105	110	0.001
Heart rate recovery in five minutes	87	98	98	103	0.001

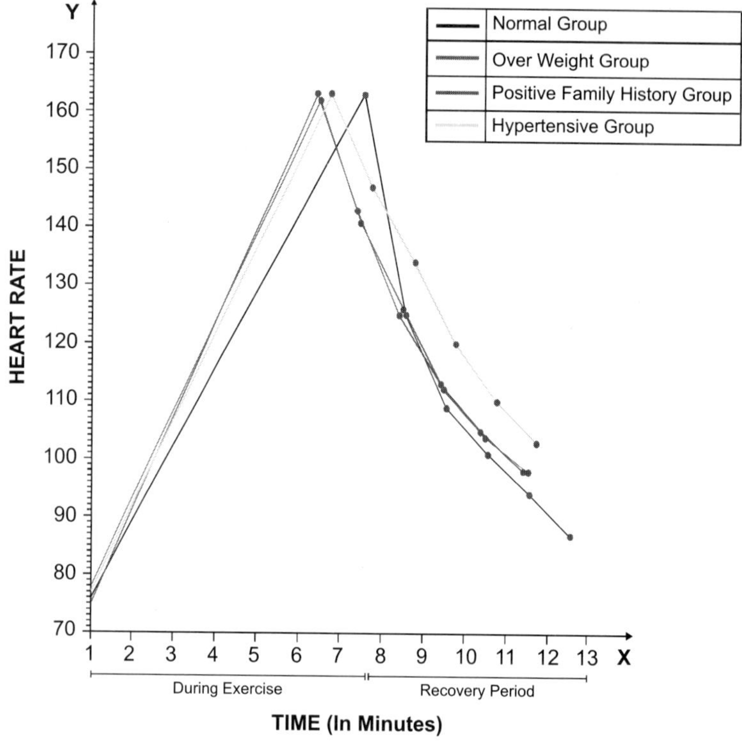

Fig. 7

fast as compare to CAD risk factors groups. Hypertensive group show slowest HRR between all the groups. (Fig. 7)

DISCUSSION

Important finding of this study is that heart rate recovery in normal group is more than coronary artery disease risk factor groups in the 1st five minutes of recovery period. In the 1st minute, heart rate recovery in normal group is approximately double than in the Coronary Artery Disease (CAD) risk factor groups as shown by results of this study.

Data from this study also shows that heart rate recovery during 2nd minute is almost same both in normal and coronary disease risk factors group. Only the overweight and hypertensive groups' show statistically significant differences i.e. heart rate recovery in hypertensive group is slower than overweight group. Results of heart rate recovery during 3rd, 4th and 5th minutes show no significant differences between normal and Coronary Artery Disease (CAD) risk factors group.

On the bases of these results, it can be stated that overall heart rate recovery mainly occurs in 1st minute as suggested by various reviewed studies and only the 1st minute of heart rate recovery can differentiate between normal and Coronary Artery Disease (CAD) risk factors groups. Results of this study are in agreement with previous researches (Imai et al,[26] Djalma.[19] Cole, Nishime, Barbara P[6,12] et. al) which proved that heart rate recovery occurs mainly in in the 1st minutes and demonstrated that 1st minutes of heart rate recovery are primary mediated by vagal reactivation, regardless of age and exercise intensity in healthy adults, In our study, 1st minutes of recovery period is the main time factor in which heart rate recovery is more in normal group as compare to Coronary Artery Disease (CAD) risk factor group.

Results of our study show that Coronary artery disease risk subjects have delayed Heart Rate Recovery (HRR) in the young age as compared with their healthy counterparts. This slow recovery indicates that Coronary Artery Disease (CAD) risk group may suffer cardiac problem in future.

On the basis of previously reviewed studies (Imai et al, Djalma.[19,26], Anthony p. Morise[17], cristopher joanny[12], Xavier Jauven,[21] Niranjan Seshadri[8], delayed heart rate recovery in our study may be due to parasympathetic system reactivation dysfunction. This parasympathetic system reactivation dysfunction may cause further complications in the future.

According to the results of our study, hypertension group shows more delayed heart rate recovery as compare to Overweight, Positive family history CAD risk factors groups. This shows that in hypertensive group, vagal reactivation dysfunctions is more as compare to overweight and positive family history group. Therefore, hypertensive group is at more risk than overweight and positive family history group. At last, we can say that Coronary Artery Disease (CAD) risk factor groups are at risk for future complication than normal group.

Based on these results, it can be stated that Heart Rate Recovery (HRR) is an important factor to be considered for evaluation of vagal function and discrimination in normal, overweight, hypertension and positive family history groups. Heart Rate Recovery (HRR) testing may be proved as valuable assessment tool to predict future cardiac problems in asymptomatic population.

CONCLUSION

This study concludes that heart rate recovery during 1st minute is an important factor to evaluation and differentiation between normal and coronary artery disease risk factors groups.

Therefore, this study concludes that, despite coronary artery disease risk factor's subjects are asymptomatic and looking healthy in young age, they have parasympathetic system dysfunction in the form of delayed HRR, which further may prove a factor for future cardiac complications in these subjects. So proper evaluation and assessment, on the bases of heart rate recovery in Coronary Artery Disease (CAD) risk factors subjects, may be helpful in physical therapy practice to reduce chances of cardiac complications at primary level. Screening of asymptomatic subjects will motivate the young individuals to reduce their CAD risk factors, reduce their body weight and reduce blood pressure by primary prevention programme in terms of regular exercises like treadmill, ergometry, aerobic exercises, walking programme, weight reduction programme, yoga, meditation etc.

References

1. J. Michael Gaziemo. Screening for coronary heart disease and its risk factor. Eugene Braunwald, & Lee Goldman MD. Primary cardiology 2nd. Edition. Elsevier science. 2003: 275-355.

2. Francesco Giallauria, Rosa Lucci, et al. Exercise based cardiac rehabilitation improves heart rate recovery in the elderly patients after myocardial infraction. The journals of gerontology series A Biological sciences and medical sciences. 2006; 61: 713-717.

3. Lynn S Bickley, MD and Peter G. Szilagyi, MD. Bates 'guide to physical examination and history taking. 9th edition: 21-66.

4. Michael Lauer, MD et al. Exercise testing in asymptomatic adults. American heart association, Inc. 2005; 112: 771-776.

5. Gibbons RJ. Abnormal heart rate recovery after exercise. Lancet. 2002; 359: 1536-1537.

6. Barbara P. Yawen MD. et al. Test Retest Reproducibility of Heart Rate Recovery after treadmill exercise. Annals of family medicine. 2003; 1: 236–241.

7. Yiling J. Cheng MD. Phd. et al. Heart Rate Recovery following maximum exercise testing as a predictor of cardio vascular disease and all cause mortality with diabetes. American Diabetes Care. 2003; 26: 2025 – 2057.

8. Niranjan Seshadri MD et. al. Association of an Abnormal Exercise HRR recovery with pulmonary function abnormalities. American College of Chest Physician. 2004; 125: 1286-1291

9. Grant D. Brinkworth, PhD; Manny Noakes, PhD et al. Weight loss improves heart rate recovery in overweight and obese men with feature of the metabolic syndrome. American Heart Journal. 2007; 152 (4): 693.

10. Vinod Raxwal MD et. al. Simple score to Diagnose coronary diseases. American College of Chest Physician. 2001; 119: 1933-1940.

11. Kai P. Savonen, et. al. Heart Rate Response during exercise test and cardiovascular mortality in middle aged men. The European Society of Cardiology. 2006; volume 27(5): 582-588.

12. Christopher R. Cole MD et. al, Heart Rate Recovery immediately after exercise as a predictor of mortality. American College of Chest Physician. 1999; Vol. 341 8): 1351-1357.

13. Erna Obenza MD,ChristopherR Cole MD et al. Heart Rate Recovery and Treadmill Exercise Score as Predictors of Mortality in Patients Referred for Exercise ECG. *JAMA*. 2000; 284: 1392-1398.

14. Katerina Shetler, MD, Rachel Marcus, MD,Victor F. Froelicher, MD et al. Heart rate recovery: validation and methodologic issues. J Am Coll Cardiol. 2001; 38: 1980-1987.

15. Morshedi-Meibodi A. et. al. Heart rate recovery after treadmill exercise testing (The Framingham heart study). Am J Cardiol. 2002 Oct. 15; 90(8): 848-52.

16. H Tsuji, FJ Venditti Jr, et al. Reduced heart rate variability and mortality risk in an elderly cohort: The Framingham Heart Study. American Heart Association. 1994; vol 90: 878-883.

17. Anthony P Morise MD, heart rate recovery. American heart association, inc. Circulation. 2004; 110: 2778-2780.

18. Lauren L. Smith, Monica Kukielka, and George E. Billman. Heart rate recovery after exercise: A predictor of ventricular fibrillation susceptibility after myocardial infarction. Am J Physiol Heart Circ Physiol. 2004; 288: 1763-1769.

19. Djalma Rabelo Ricardo Ph.D. et. al. Initial and final Exercise Transients. Chest medicine. 2005; 127: 318-327.

20. Prof. Guido Grassi et al. Sympathetic activation and prognosis in cardiovascular disease. E-Journal. 2007; vol. 5.

21. Xavier Jouven MD Phd. et al. Heart Rate Profiles during exercise as a predictor of sudden death. The new England Journal of Medicine. 2005; Vol – 352(9): 1951 – 1995.

22. Curfman GD, Hillis LD. A new look at cardiac exercise testing. N Engl J Med. 2003; 348: 775-776.

23. Jeffrey J. Goldberger, Francis Kiet Le, Marc Lahiri. Assessment of parasympathetic reactivation after exercise. Am J Physiol Heart Circ Physiol. 2006; 290: 2446-2452.

24. Sammy Gammenthaler, M.D. Recovery of Heart Rate after Exercise. New England journal of medicine. 2002 ; Volume 342(9): 662-663.

25. Victor F. Froelicher, Jonathan Myers. Exercise and the Heart. 5th edition 2006. Elsevier Inc: 36-37, 113-114.

26. Imai K, Sato H, Hori M, et al. Vagal mediated heart rate recovery after exercise is accelerated in athletes but blunted in patients with chronic heart failure. J Am Coll Cardiol. 1994; 24: 1529-1535.

27. Fredric J. Pashkow, MD & William A. Dafoe, MD. Clinical Cardiac Rehabilitation : A Cardiologists Guide. 2nd. Edition. 1999: 65-101

13

Effect of Training on Physiological and Biochemical Variables of Indian Football Players of Various Age Groups

I. Manna[a, c], G.L. Khanna[b] and P.C. Dhara[c]

[a]Department of Physiology, Janaki Medical College, Janakpur, Nepal
[b]Department of Health Sciences, Manav Rachana Educational Institute, Faridabad, India
[c]Department of Human Physiology, Vidyasagar University, Midnapore, India

ABSTRACT

Football is the most popular sports worldwide. The present study is aimed to find out the effect of training on physiological and biochemical variables of Indian football players of various age groups. A total of one handed and twenty (N = 120) male football players volunteered for the present study. The players were divided into 4 groups (n = 30): under 16 years (14-16 yrs), under 19 years (16-18 yrs), under 23 years (19-22 yrs), and senior (23-30 yrs). The training sessions were divided into 3 phases: [transition phase (TP), 4 weeks], [preparatory phase (PP), 8 weeks], and [competitive phase (CP), 4 weeks]. The training programme consisted of aerobic, anaerobic and skill training; and completed 4 hours in morning and evening sessions, 5 days/week. Different physiological and biochemical parameters were tested at each training phase using standard measuring technique and data were analyzed by applying two-way ANOVA and post hoc test. The results showed increase ($P < 0.05$) in VO_{2max}, anaerobic power, strength, urea, uric acid and high density lipoprotein (HDL); and on the other hand , decrease ($P < 0.05$) in body fat, haemoglobin (Hb), total cholesterol (TC), triglyceride (TG) and low density lipoprotein (LDL) has been observed in PP and CP when compared with TP. Moreover, the differences in the above parameters from PP to CP were found to be negligible. Further, a significant increase ($P < 0.05$) in height, weight, VO_{2max}, anaerobic power, strength, Hb, urea, uric acid, TC, TG, HDL and LDL and a decrease ($P < 0.05$) in body fat has been observed in the senior players when compared to that of the juniors. These changes may be due to alterations in volume and intensities of training in different training phases. Long term exposure to training and maturation make the difference between the senior and junior players. The present study will provide useful information about training and selection of football players of different age categories.

1.0 INTRODUCTION

Football (soccer) is unarguably the world's most popular sport. The common aspect of the game is the necessity of teamwork to complement individual skills. Since football is a physical contact sport and lots of movements and skills are involved. A high level of physical demand is required for match play, which involves kicking, short sprinting, throwing, catching, trapping etc. The activities of the game include short sprinting as well as casual recovery movements. As the players have to cover a big area in the ground during attack and defense therefore, the game demands for aerobic as well as anaerobic fitness [1, 2]. To achieve the best possible performance in football the training has to be formulated according to the principles of periodization [3]. In its simplest form "periodization of training "means" dividing the training up into periods" [3]. The training induced changes observed in various physiological and biochemical variables can be attributed to incremental training load [3]. This would enable the coaches to assess the current status of an athlete and the degree of training adaptability and provide an opportunity to modify the training schedule accordingly to achieve the desired performance [3]. Apart from the skills and teamwork required for game play body composition; strength, aerobic capacity and anaerobic power as well as heart rate during exercise and recovery have significant impact [4-7]. Moreover, biochemical profiles like hemoglobin; urea, uric acid, lipids and lipoproteins are also good indicators for monitoring of training and physical fitness [8-11]. The present study has been focused on football players as the performance of the Indian football team is very limited at the international level, and there is limited research work available in India o the effect of training on football players. The purpose of the investigation was to conduct a study of physiological and biochemical variables among Indian football players with reference to age and training.

2.0 METHODOLOGY

2.1 Subjects

A total of one hundred and twenty (N = 120) male players, regularly playing competitive football, volunteered for the present study were selected from the National training camps at Sports Authority of India. The players were divided into 4 groups (n = 30): under 16 years (14-16 yrs); under 19 years (16-18 yrs); under 23 years (19-22 yrs); and senior (23-30 yrs). The training sessions were divided into 3 phases: [transition phase (TP), 4 weeks], [preparatory phase (PP), 8 weeks], and [competitive phase (CP), 4 weeks]. The training programme consisted of aerobic, anaerobic and skill training; and completed

4 hours in morning and evening sessions, 5 days/week. Physiological and biochemical variables were measured in the laboratory. Each test was scheduled at the same time of day (± 1 hour) in order to minimize the effect of diurnal variation. All the experiments were performed at 25 ± 1°C, with relative humidity of 60 - 65%. A written informed consent was taken from all the participants, about the possible comlpicaions of the study.

2.2   Measurement of Physiological Parameters

Body mass was measured with the accurately calibrated electronic scale (Seca Alpha 770, UK) to the nearest 0.1 kg and height with a stadiometer (Seca 220, UK) recorded to the nearest 0.1 cm [12]. Percent body fat was derived from skin folds taken from various sites of the body and using a standard equation [13]. Lean body mass (LBM) was calculated by subtracting fat mass from total body mass. Grip and back strength were measured by dynamometers (Senoh, Japan) [12]. Maximal aerobic capacity (VO_{2max}) and heart rate during exercise and recovery were measured using treadmill and metabolic analyzer (Jaeger, Germany) following standard methodology [14]. Anaerobic power was measured using a cycle ergometer (Jaeger, Germany) following a standard procedure [15].

2.3   Measurement of Biochemical Parameters

A 5 ml of venous blood was drawn from an antecubital vein after a 12 hour fast and 24 hour after the last bout of exercise. Haemoglobin (Hb) [16] urea [17] and uric acid [18] were measured following standard methodology. Total cholesterol (TC) [19], triglyceride (TG) [20] and high-density lipoprotein (HDL) [19] were determined by enzymatic method using standard methodology. Low-density lipoprotein (LDL) was derived indirectly from the equation of Friedewald et al [21]. All the reagents were procured form a reliable company.

2.4   Statistical Analysis

Data were presented as mean and standard deviation. Two-way ANOVA followed by Post hoc test was used to determine whether the differences of means in each parameter were significant. Differences were considered significant when $P < 0.05$. Accordingly, a statistical software package (SPSS) was used.

3.0   RESULTS & DISCUSSION

In the present study no significant difference has been observed in height and body mass among the football players after the training programme. It may be due to the shorter duration of the training or due to improper optimization of the training load. However, differences ($p < 0.05$) have been observed in height and body mass among the players of different age categories. It has been observed that long term exercise training has significant effect on height and body mass [22]. Therefore, increase in height and body mass from junior to senior level was observed. The gain in height and body mass is dependent on growth hormone and exercise is a potent stimulus for growth hormone [23]. The percent body fat of all the players decreased ($p < 0.05$) during the preparatory and competitive phases of training when compared with transition phase in the present study. The reduction in body fat may be due to the fact that the sportsmen are undergoing high intensity and volume of training over a period of time, which results in lowering of body fat percentage. The possible reason of reduction of body fat is endurance training which increases greater utilization of fat for energetic [24]. The percentage body fat also decreased ($p < 0.05$) with the advancement of age of the players. On the other hand, LBM ($p < 0.05$) increased with the advancement of age of the players. The low body fat values in the senior players may be because of exposure to higher amount of aerobic endurance training compared with juniors.

Table 3.1 Effect of training on height, body mass, body fat and LBM of football players of different age groups

Parameters	Training phase	Age group			
		U16	U19	U23	SR
Height (cm)	TP	166.8 ± 4.2	171.7* ± 4.7	173.8*# ± 4.5	174.6*# ± 3.6
	PP	166.9 ± 4.2	171.7* ± 4.7	173.8*# ± 4.6	174.6*# ± 3.6
	CP	166.9 ± 4.1	171.7* ± 4.7	173.9*# ± 4.7	174.6*# ± 3.6
Body mass (kg)	TP	52.8 ± 1.3	58.9* ± 4.9	64.7*# ± 5.0	65.3*# ± 5.9
	PP	51.7 ± 1.7	57.7* ± 4.6	63.1*# ± 5.0	64.3*# ± 6.0
	CP	51.1 ± 1.7	57.1* ± 4.6	63.0*# ± 5.2	64.0*# ± 6.3
Body fat (%)	TP	16.6 ± 2.0	14.3*‡ ± 2.3	13.9*#‡ ± 2.2	12.7*#¥‡ ± 2.7
	PP	15.0‡ ± 2.7	13.4*‡ ± 2.9	12.1*#‡ ± 2.2	12.0*#¥‡ ± 2.6
	CP	15.0‡ ± 2.1	13.0*‡ ± 1.3	12.1*#‡ ± 1.5	12.0*#¥‡ ± 2.2
LBM (kg)	TP	40.8 ± 1.8	47.1*‡ ± 4.1	51.3*# ± 4.3	53.1*# ± 4.9
	PP	41.1 ± 2.4	48.3*‡ ± 4.1	52.5*# ± 4.4	53.9*# ± 5.2
	CP	41.1 ± 2.8	48.7*‡ ± 4.4	52.7*# ± 4.4	53.9*# ± 5.5

Data presented as mean ± SD; n = 30; $P < 0.05$; * when compared to U16, # when compared to U19, ¥ when compared to U23, ‡ when compared to TP, U16 = under 16 yrs, U19 = under 19 yrs, U23 = under 23 yrs, SR = senior age groups; TP = transition phase, PP = preparatory phase, CP = competitive phase; LBM = lean body mass.

In the present study significant increase ($p < 0.05$) in VO_{2max} has been noted in Under 16 years and Under 19 years football players in the preparatory phase when compared with transition phase. This may be because of the increase volume of endurance training in preparatory phase. Further, a decline in VO_{2max} values has been observed, although non-significantly, from preparatory phase to competitive phase, which may be because of the reduction in aerobic training in competitive phase. On the other hand, no significant change has been noted in VO_{2max} values of the Under 23 years and senior age group players after the training programme. It can be suggested that VO_{2max} of the football players improve with training and the improvement is higher in the junior players than seniors. The VO_{2max} also elevates ($p < 0.05$) during adolescence and then declines ($p < 0.05$) in the senior age group players in the present study. It has been found that the junior players possess similar mean relative VO_{2max} values as the senior players. This lower mean VO_{2max} values in the senior players may be due to their higher body mass [24, 25]. It is suggested that percentage fat, training hours and motivation influence this development. Training has no significant change in maximal heart rate but recovery heart rate decreases ($p < 0.05$) after training among the players. The maximal and recovery heart rate also decreases ($p < 0.05$) as the players become mature.

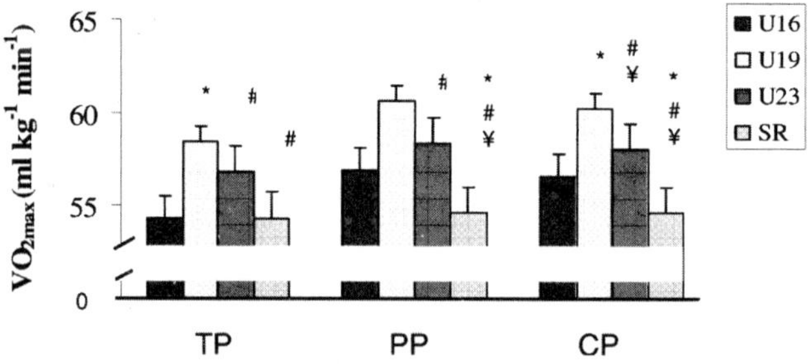

Fig. 3.1 VO_{2max} of football players of different age group
Data presented as mean and SD, n = 30; P < 0.05; Data were significantly different from each other when compared to (U16 *P < 0.050, U19 # P < 0.050, U23 ¥P < 0.050); U16 = under 16 yrs, U19 = under 19 yrs, U23 = under 23 yrs, SR = senior age groups; TP = transition phase, PP = preparatory phase, CP = competitive phase.

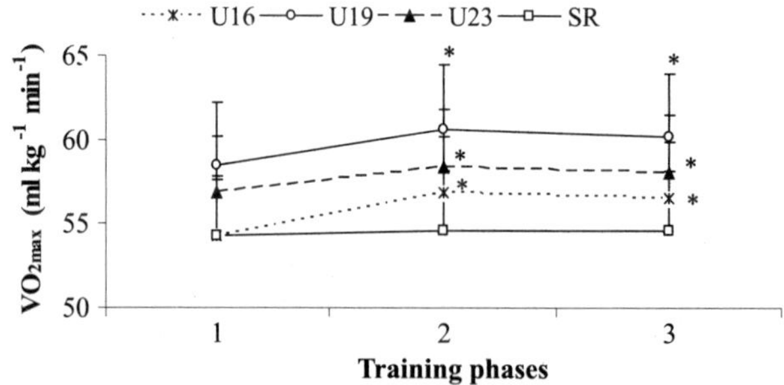

Fig. 3.2   Effect of training on VO_{2max} of football players
Data presented as mean and SD, n = 30; P < 0.05; Data were significantly different from each other when compared to (1 *P < 0.050, 2 #P < 0.050); U16 = under 16 yrs, U19 = under 19 yrs, U23 = under 23 yrs, SR = senior age groups; 1 = transition phase, 2 = preparatory phase, 3 = competitive phase.

Table 3.2 Effect of training on heart rate and strength of football players of different age groups

Parameters	Training phase	Age group			
		U16	U19	U23	SR
Maximal heart rate (beats min^{-1})	TP	193.8 ± 3.7	189.5* ± 3.5	185.5$^{*\#}$ ± 3.4	181.7$^{*\#}$ ± 4.6
	PP	193.2 ± 5.6	188.0* ± 4.9	184.4$^{*\#}$ ± 5.6	181.3$^{*\#}$ ± 5.4
	CP	193.3 ± 5.1	188.1* ± 5.7	184.0$^{*\#}$ ± 5.5	181.0$^{*\#}$ ± 4.1
Recovery heart rate (beats min^{-1})	TP	162.7 ± 4.8	155.8* ± 4.6	154.9$^{*\#\ddagger}$ ± 3.6	151.6$^{*\#\ddagger}$ ± 3.3
	PP	159.3‡ ± 4.9	151.9*‡ ± 3.8	150.3$^{*\#\ddagger}$ ± 4.4	148.7$^{*\#\ddagger}$ ± 4.7
	CP	160.3‡ ± 4.9	151.9*‡ ± 4.3	150.6$^{*\#\ddagger}$ ± 4.2	149.2$^{*\#\ddagger}$ ± 4.7
Back strength (kg)	TP	105.7 ± 4.2	112.2* ± 4.7	118.9$^{*\#}$ ± 3.1	124.2$^{*\#}$ ± 4.6
	PP	107.0‡ ± 4.2	114.5*‡ ± 4.5	122.5$^{*\#\ddagger}$ ± 4.5	125.4$^{*\#\ddagger}$ ± 4.5
	CP	107.8‡ ± 4.3	114.6*‡ ± 4.9	123.3$^{*\#\ddagger}$ ± 4.9	125.8$^{*\#\ddagger}$ ± 3.0
Grip strength of right hand (kg)	TP	27.6 ± 3.3	31.2* ± 3.8	36.2$^{*\#}$ ± 3.4	39.8$^{*\#}$ ± 3.5
	PP	29.0‡ ± 3.9	33.1*‡ ± 3.4	39.9$^{*\#\ddagger}$ ± 3.5	40.0$^{*\#\ddagger}$ ± 3.8
	CP	29.1‡ ± 3.7	33.3*‡ ± 3.2	37.8$^{*\#\ddagger}$ ± 4.0	40.5$^{*\#\ddagger}$ ± 3.3
Grip strength of left hand (kg)	TP	26.6 ± 3.9	30.5* ± 2.8	33.9$^{*\#}$ ± 3.6	35.3$^{*\#}$ ± 3.5
	PP	29.3‡ ± 3.2	32.2*‡ ± 3.8	35.5$^{*\#\ddagger}$ ± 3.7	36.8$^{*\#\ddagger}$ ± 3.4
	CP	29.5‡ ± 3.2	32.6*‡ ± 3.2	35.9$^{*\#\ddagger}$ ± 3.9	36.6$^{*\#\ddagger}$ ± 3.3

Data presented as mean ± SD; n = 30; P < 0.05; * when compared to U16, # when compared to U19, ¥ when compared to U23, ‡ when compared to TP, U16 = under 16 yrs, U19 = under 19 yrs, U23 = under 23 yrs, SR = senior age groups; TP = transition phase, PP = preparatory phase, CP = competitive phase.

The strength of back and grip; and anaerobic power increased (p < 0.05) after the training programme among the players in the present study. It can be sated that as the training load increases from transition phase to preparatory and competitive phase, the players involved in more of strength and power training which results in an increase in these parameters [1, 2, 24]. Further, in the present study increase (p < 0.05) in strength, and anaerobic power have also been noted with the advancement of age of the players. The above age related increase in strength and power may be due to the increase body mass

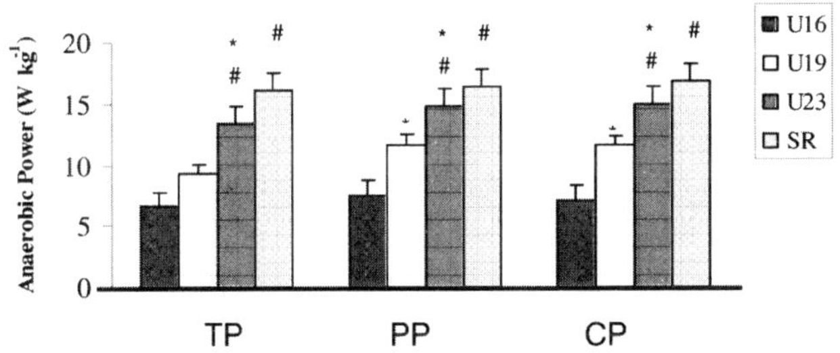

Fig. 3.3 Anaerobic power of Indian football players of different age group

Data presented as mean and SD, n = 30; P < 0.05; Data were significantly different from each other when compared to (U16 *P < 0.050, U19 # P < 0.050, U23 ¥P < 0.050); U16 = under 16 yrs, U19 = under 19 yrs, U23 = under 23 yrs, SR = senior age groups; TP = transition phase, PP = preparatory phase, CP = competitive phase.

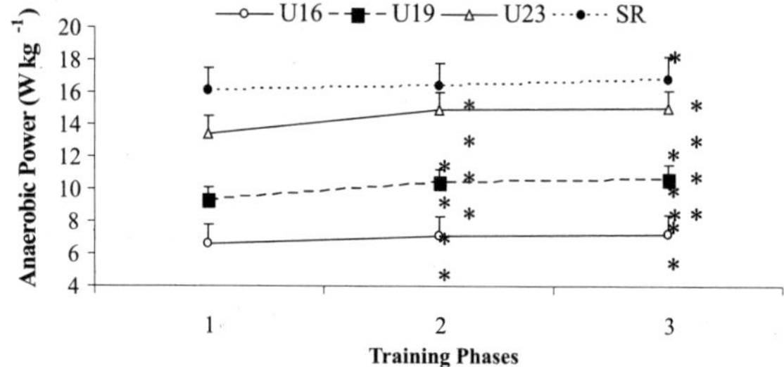

Fig. 3.4 Effect of training on anaerobic power of Indian football players
Data presented as mean and SD, n = 30; $P < 0.05$; Data were significantly different from each other when compared to (1 * $P < 0.050$, 2 # $P < 0.050$); U16 = under 16 yrs, U19 = under 19 yrs, U23 = under 23 yrs, SR = senior age groups; 1 = transition phase, 2 = preparatory phase, 3 = competitive phase.

throughout the developmental process and also due to the neural recruitment. It can be suggested that as the age of the sportsmen increases, they gradually undergo more strength and power training, which helps to increase muscle mass resulting in improving strength and power component.

Table 3.3 Effect of training on haemoglobin, serum urea, uric acid, triglyceride and LDL levels of football players of different age groups

Parameters	Training phase	Age group			
		U16	U19	U23	SR
Haemoglobin (gm dl⁻¹)	TP	13.7 ± 0.5	14.0 ± 0.6	14.4*# ± 0.5	14.5*#¥ ± 0.6
	PP	13.5 ± 0.6	13.6‡ ± 0.6	14.1*# ± 0.8	14.3*#¥‡ ± 0.7
	CP	13.4 ± 0.6	13.6‡ ± 0.6	14.0*#‡ ± 0.7	14.1*#¥‡ ± 0.6
Urea (mg dl⁻¹)	TP	22.7 ± 2.0	27.1* ± 2.7	28.1*# ± 2.8	29.3*#¥ ± 2.3
	PP	23.1‡ ± 2.0	28.0*‡ ± 3.0	29.2*#‡ ± 2.3	30.4*#¥‡ ± 2.5
	CP	27.8‡ ± 2.7	31.3*‡† ± 2.9	32.1*#‡† ± 2.5	32.1*#¥‡ ± 2.2
Uric acid (mg dl⁻¹)	TP	3.1 ± 0.3	3.5 ± 0.5	4.2*# ± 0.6	4.1*# ± 0.5
	PP	3.4 ± 0.2	3.9 ± 0.5	4.5*# ± 0.6	4.3*# ± 0.5
	CP	3.7 ± 0.2	3.9‡ ± 0.6	4.8*#‡ ± 0.6	4.6*#‡ ± 0.5
Triglyceride (mg dl⁻¹)	TP	58.6 ± 4.3	64.9 ± 5.5	87.9*# ± 5.2	104.1*#¥ ± 6.1
	PP	56.4 ± 4.9	62.7 ± 5.7	85.1*#‡ ± 5.7	102.4*#¥ ± 6.2
	CP	55.8 ± 5.2	62.2 ± 5.7	84.7*#‡ ± 5.1	101.3*#¥‡ ± 6.8
LDL (mg dl⁻¹)	TP	99.4 ± 5.1	102.4* ± 5.3	100.4*# ± 4.1	105.5*#¥ ± 5.6
	PP	97.6 ± 5.4	101.0*‡ ± 4.8	99.0*# ± 5.4	103.4*#¥ ± 5.4
	CP	96.7 ± 5.3	100.0*‡ ± 4.3	98.2*# ± 5.9	103.1*#¥ ± 5.2

Data presented as mean ± SD; n = 30; $P < 0.05$; * when compared to U16, # when compared to U19, ¥ when compared to U23, ‡ when compared to TP, † when compared to PP; U16 = under 16 yrs, U19 = under 19 yrs, U23 = under 23 yrs, SR = senior age groups; TP = transition phase, PP = preparatory phase, CP = competitive phase; LDL = low density lipoprotein.

The haemoglobin level decreased ($p < 0.05$) after training programme among all the players in the present study. During transition phase the training load is less than preparatory phase and competitive phase, therefore in the preparatory phase and competitive phase reduced haemoglobin level has been observed. This decline in haemoglobin level may be due to haemolysis [26]. Further, exercise-induced haemolysis may be due to oxidative stress in exercising muscles [27]. However, the level of haemoglobin increased ($p < 0.05$) with the advancement of age of the player. The present study shows that the haemoglobin level increases as the players become mature. This might be due to the higher body size of the senior players than the juniors. It can be stated that body mass and VO_{2max} increases with the advancement of age of the players. The increase in VO_{2max} demands higher rate of supply of oxygen, which is transported to muscle primarily by haemoglobin. Therefore, it is suggested that haemoglobin mass and/or concentration is related to VO_{2max} [21, 24].

The level of serum urea and urea acid increased after training among the players in the present study. It has been observed that as the training load

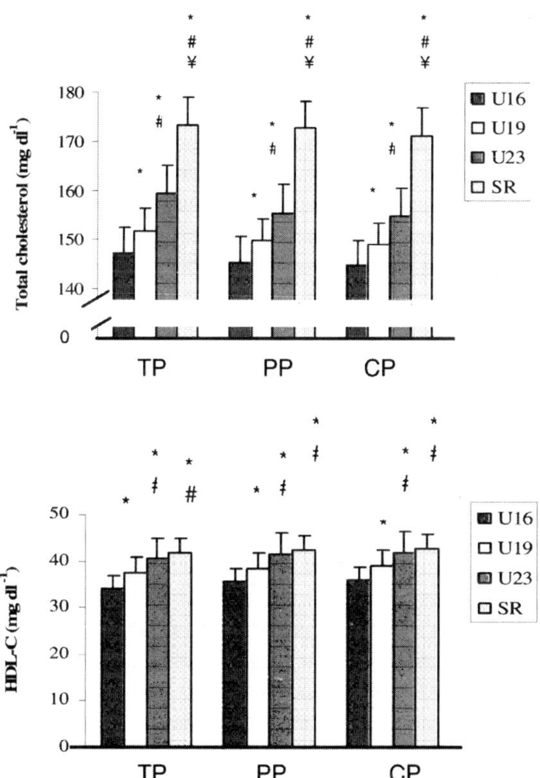

Fig. 3.5 Total Cholesterol and HDL of Indian football players of different age group

Data presented as mean and SD, n = 30; P < 0.05; Data were significantly different from each other when compared to (U16 * P < 0.050, U19 # P < 0.050, U23 ¥ P < 0.050); U16 = under 16 yrs, U19 = under 19 yrs, U23 = under 23 yrs, SR = senior age groups; TP = transition phase, PP = preparatory phase, CP = competitive phase.

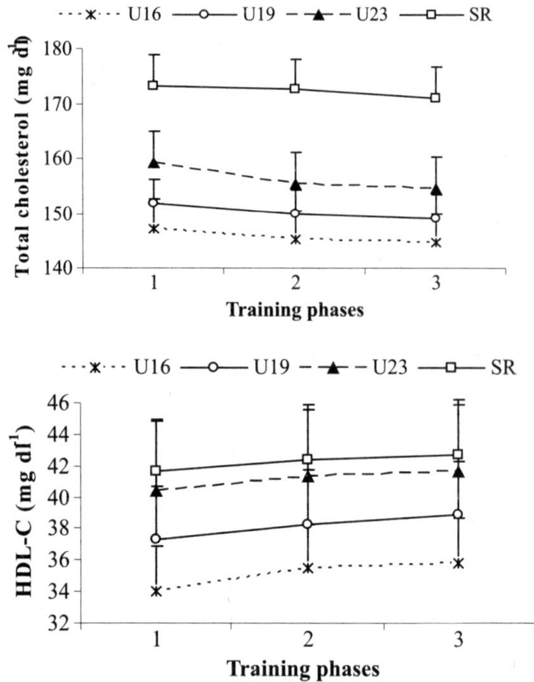

Fig. 3.6 Effect of training on Total Cholesterol and HDL of Indian football players

Data presented as mean and SD, n = 30; P < 0.05; Data were significantly different from each other when compared to (1 * P < 0.050, 2 # P < 0.050); U16 = under 16 yrs, U19 = under 19 yrs, U23 = under 23 yrs, SR = senior age groups; 1 = transition phase, 2 = preparatory phase, 3 = competitive phase.

increases, from transition phase to preparatory phase and in the competitive phase, the urea and uric acid level increased gradually. It is believed that a pronounced increase in the urea and uric acid concentration indicates strong influence of a training session, whereas normalization of the urea and uric acid level in blood is an index of time to perform subsequent strenuous training sessions. The possible reason for the increased urea level is the breakdown of proteins; where as increase in uric acid level after the training programme might be due to oxidative damage to exercising muscles [7, 28]. The level of serum urea and uric acid also increased (p < 0.05) with the advancement of age of the players in the present study. This higher urea and uric acid level might be due to increased training load or high amount of protein intake in the senior players when compared with the juniors [7, 28].

Activity levels have significant impact on the lipids and lipoprotein levels of the athletes. In the present study, decrease (p < 0.05) in total cholesterol, triglyceride and LDL level; and increase (p < 0.05) in HDL level has been noted among the players after the training programme. It can be stated that increased physical activity induces a number of positive changes in the metabolism of lipids and lipoproteins [6, 29]. In the present study increased (p < 0.050) levels of total cholesterol, triglyceride, HDL and LDL level have also been observed with the advancement of age of the players. It indicated that maturation process has positive relationship with the lipids and lipoproteins levels of the athletes. It has been reported that cholesterol and LDL has the greatest correlation to severity of coronary atherosclerosis [6, 29]. Therefore, monitoring of lipid profile in athletes can provide valuable information about their metabolic and cardiovascular status.

CONCLUSION

In the present study, training induced changes in different physiological and biochemical parameters have been noted in Indian football players of different age categories. It may be concluded that training improve the aerobic, anaerobic and strength components of the players. These changes were reflected on various physiological and biochemical variables like body fat, haemoglobin, urea, uric acid, and lipid profile. As the studies on football players are limited in India, the present study may provide a useful database to the coaches for monitoring of training schedules.

References

1. Reilly T (1996) *Science and soccer* E & FN Spon, London.
2. Reilly T, Bangsbo J and Ranks A (2000a): Anthropometric and physiological predisposition for elite soccer. *J. Sport. Sci.,* 18, 669-683.
3. Bompa TO. Periodization Training for Sports. Champaign, IL, Human Kinetics, 1999.
4. Aziz AR, Chia M and The KC (2000): The relationship between maximal oxygen uptake and repeated sprint performance indices in field hockey and soccer players. *J. Sport. Med. Phys. Fit.,* 40, 195-200.
5. Carraro, F., Kimbrough, T. D. and Wolfe, R. R., 1993. Urea kinetics in humans of two levels of exercise intensity. J. Applied Physiology 75, 1180-1185.
6. Chin MK, So RC, Yuan YW, Li RC and Wong AS (1994): Cardio respiratory fitness and isokinetic muscle strength of elite Asian soccer players. *J. Sport. Med. Phys. Fit.,* 34, 250-257.
7. Urhausen A and Kindermann W (2002): Diagnosis of over training: what tools do we have? *Sport. Med.,* 32, 95-102.
8. Berg, A., Frey, I., Basmstark, M. W., Halle, M. and Keul, J., 1994. Physical activity and lipoprotein lipid disorders. Sports Medicine 17, 6-21.
9. Casoni, I., Barsetto, C., Cavicchi, A., Martinelli, S. and Conconi, F., 1985. Reduced hemoglobin concentration and red cells hemoglobinization in Italian marathon and ultra marathon runners. Int. J. Sports Medicine 6, 176-179.
10. Cerny F (1975): Protein metabolism during two hours ergometer exercise. In: *Metabolic adaptation to prolonged physical exercise* (H. Howald and J. R. Poortmans, eds.) Birkhauser, Basel, p. 232-237.
11. Fry RW, Morton AR, Garcia-Webb P and Keast D (1991): Monitoring exercise stress by changes in metabolic and hormonal responses over a 24-h period. *Eu. J. Appl. Physiol. Occup. Physiol.,* 63, 228-234.

12. Jonson, B. L. and Nelson, J. K., 1996. Practical measurements for evaluation in physical education. London: Macmillan Publishing Co.

13. Siri, W. E., 1956. The gross composition of the body. In C. A. Tobias and J. H. Lawrence (Ed.), Advances in Biological and Medical Physics. (pp. 239-280). New York: Academic Press.

14. Astrand, P. O. and Rodhal, K., 1970. Textbook of work physiology. New York: McGraw-Hill.

15. Inbar, O., Bar-Or, O. and Skinner, J. S., 1996. The Wingate anaerobic test. Champaign IL: Human Kinetics.

16. Mukharjee, K. L., 1997. Medical laboratory technology. A procedure manual for routine diagnostic tests. Vol I - III., New Delhi: Tata McGraw-Hill Publishing Company Limited.

17. Wybenga D R, Di Giorgio J and Pileggi VJ. Manual and automated methods for urea nitrogen measurement in whole serum. *Clin Chem* 1971; 17: 891-5.

18. Martinek RG. Review of methods for determining inorganic phosphorus in biological fluids. *J Am Med Technol* 1970; 32: 237.

19. Wybenga D R, Pileggi VJ, Dirstine PH and Di Giorgio J. Direct manual determination of serum total cholesterol with a single stable reagent. *Clin Chem* 1970; 16: 980-4.

20. Schettler G and Nussei E. Ma?nahmen zur Prävention der Arteriosklerose. *Arb Med Soz Med Prav Med* 1975; 10: 25.

21. Friedewald, W. T., Levy, R.I. and Fredrickson, D. S., 1972. Estimation of the concentration of low density lipoprotein cholesterol in plasma without use of the preparative ultracentrifuge. Clinical Chemistry 18, 499-501.

22. Wilmore JH and Costill DL. *Physiology of Sport and Exercise: 3rd Edition.* Champaign IL, Human Kinetics, 2005.

23. Coyel EF, Hemmert MK, Coggan AR, *et al.* Effect of detraining on cardiovascular responses to exercise: role of blood volume. *J Appl Physiol* 1986; 60: 95-9.

24. Mc Ardle WD, Katch FI and Katch VL. Essentials of Exercise Physiology: 3rd ed. Philadelphia PA, Lippincott Williams & Wilkins, 2006.

25. Reilly T. An Ergonomics model of the soccer training process. *J Sports Sci* 2005; 6: 561-572.

26. Boning D, Klarholz C, Himmelsbach B, Hutler M and Maassen N. Extracellular bicarbonate and non-bicarbonate buffering against lactic acid during and after exercise. *Eur J Appl Physiol* 2007; 100: 457-67.

27. Senturk UK, Gunduz F, Kuru O, Kocer G, Ozkaya YG, Yesilkaya A, Bor-Kucukatay M, Uyuklu M, Yalcin O and Baskurt OK. Exercise-induced oxidative stress leads hemolysis in sedentary but not trained humans. *J Appl Physiol* 2005; 99:1434-41.

28. Tsahar E, Arad Z, Izhaki I and Guglielmo CG. The relationship between uric acid and its oxidative product allantoin: a potential indicator for the evaluation of oxidative stress in birds. *J Comp Physiol* 2006; 176: 653-61.

29. Durstine JL, Davis PG, Ferguson MA, Alderson NL and Trost SG. Effects of short-duration and long-duration exercise on lipoprotein (a). *Med Sci Sports Exerc* 2001; 33: 1511-6.

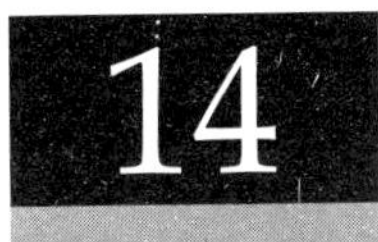

Critical Power Testing in Acute Hypobaric Hypoxia

K.K. Tripathi[1]*, A. Chawla[2], S.S. Mishra[3] and P. Kharbanda[4]

[1]SMO & Senior Advisor in Aviation Medicine, Air Force Station, Adampur
Jalandhar - 144 103 Punjab
[2]Classified Specialist, High Altitude Medical Research Centre, 153 GH, C/O 56 APO
[3]Classified Specialist (Physiology)
Defence Institute of Physiology & Allied Sciences, Timarpur, Delhi - 110 054
[4]Deputy Principal Medical Officer & Senior Advisor (Aviation Medicine)
HQ WAC, IAF, Subroto Park, New Delhi - 110 010

ABSTRACT

Critical power (CP) and anaerobic work capacity (AWC) were measured in a group of 14 healthy, male, untrained, non smokers at ground level (3159' above msl) and two altitudes (i.e. 6000 ft and 10000 ft) simulated in a hypobaric chamber. Subjects performed four dynamic work tests (with power loadings 200, 225, 250 and 275 watts) up to the onset of muscular fatigue in the maximum time (T_{Limit}) beyond which the initial power output levels could no longer be maintained. The total work performed (W_{Limit}) was defined as the product of the imposed power loading P and the T_{Limit}. CP and AWC were derived as slope coefficient (b) and Y-intercept (a), respectively, of the line defined by the relationship between W_{Limit} and T_{Limit}. Between two such exercise bouts, subjects recovered in normoxia. PWC170 was also measured with a separate incremental exercise protocol. No significant effect of altitude was noted on AWC (F = 0.98; p = 0.388). However, CP decreased significantly, from its ground level value of 136 ± 5 watts, to 115 ± 8 watts at 6000 ft and 96 ± 7 watts at 10,000 ft (F = 13.5; p = 0.000). The above change represented a reduction of about 15 ± 5% at 6,000 ft and 28 ± 6% at 10,000 ft. CP accounted for 98 ± 4% of PWC170 at ground level. It declined significantly (F = 13.1; p = 0.000) to 81 ± 4% and 68 ± 4% at 6000 ft and 10000 ft, respectively. Within this altitude range,

---

Corresponding Author

CP could be regressed as CP (in watts) = 137 − 4, altitude (in 1,000 ft) (F = 15.75, p < 0.0003 & SE of estimate = 2.42). Susceptibility of CP to hypoxia and invariance of AWC during hypoxia submits an indirect support to CP theory.

INTRODUCTION

Concept of critical power (CP) was originally proposed by Monod & Scherrer (1965) for synergistic muscle groups. In experiments in which a small muscle group worked at different constant rates till muscular exhaustion, these authors observed a linear relationship between the total work done at each rate and its duration. The slope of this relation was termed 'critical power' and was considered to represent the power output that a muscle group could maintain without exhaustion. A cycle ergometer analogue of the CP test was developed by Moritani et al (1981). Evaluation of CP involves a series of exhaustive work bouts at various power loadings from which the total amount of work performed or work limit (W_{Limit}) and the time to exhaustion or time limit (T_{Lim}) are determined. The W_{Limit} is defined as the product of the imposed power loading P and the T_{Limit} (ie, $W_{Limit} = P \cdot T_{Limit}$). The relationship between W_{Limit} and T_{Limit} is given by the equation for a straight line:

$$W_{Limit} = a + b \, (T_{Limit})$$

The slope (b) and Y-intercept (a) of the W_{Limit} versus T_{Limit} plot have been termed critical power (CP) and anaerobic work capacity (AWC) respectively. It has been suggested that CP represents the rate of energy supply, magnitude of which determines the maximal power at which a muscle can work without fatigue whereas AWC represents both the energy contained in the high energy phosphorous compounds and that originating from the use of intramuscular glycogen and is independent of circulatory oxygen supply.

Attempts have been made for experimental validation of CP theory. These include: **1)** association of CP and AWC with endurance and strength status and/or conditioning, **2)** their comparison with other indicators of aerobic and anaerobic capacities and finally, endorsement of their susceptibility/ insusceptibility to certain experimental manipulations like dietary creatine supplementation, hypoxia etc. Certain studies (Tripathi & Banerjee, 1991) have shown that trained subjects possess significantly higher values of CP compared to untrained. Specific susceptibility of CP & AWC to endurance (Gaesser & Wilson 1988; Jenkins & Quigley 1992) and strength (Jenkins & Quigley 1993) conditioning support the aerobic and anaerobic nature of the CP and AWC respectively. Additionally, CP and AWC have been shown to be related to other measures of aerobic and anaerobic performance/capacity. For instance, Moritani et al (1981) and deVries et al (1987) found CP to be highly correlated with **Anaerobic Threshold** (AT) and **Physical Work Capacity at fatigue threshold** (PWCFT). As a matter of fact, Moritani et al (1981) found almost identical values of CP and AT. Similarly, Jenkins & Quigley (1991) noted a significant relation between the y-intercept (from the critical power curve) and total work accomplished. Hill & Smith (1993) further validated y-intercept as a measure of anaerobic capacity, using maximal oxygen deficit as the criterion measure. In this study, individual AWC were calculated by nonlinear regression of time with power, with time as the dependent variable. Oxygen deficit was determined during each bout, and the mean of the values obtained from the power output which elicited the highest values was used as the criterion for anaerobic capacity. The estimates of AWC and criterion measures were the same. Dietary supplementation with creatine increases AWC (Smith et al. 1998; Miura et al. 1999; Stout et al. 1999).

CP testing in a hypoxic environment constitutes a unique experimental manipulation to examine the robustness of the theory which permits one to hypothesise a marked reduction in CP and an invariance of AWC during short term exposure to hypoxia. Nevertheless, such an approach has hardly been made to evaluate CP testing procedure. Except for a limited (albeit first of its kind) effort by Moritani et al (1981), we could not find any study which tested CP and AWC in hypoxia. In their study, Moritani et al. (1981) examined effects of acute normobaric hypoxia on CP and AWC in two subjects and reported a decrease in CP from 197 watts while breathing 20.9% to 110 watts while breathing 9.0% oxygen. The corresponding values in the second subject were 230 watt and 102 watts, respectively. Intercept was unaffected. The AWC values are not given in the article. However, it appears, from Fig. 6 of Moritani et al (1981) that AWC was a little more than 200 watt. min for the first subject and a little less than 400 watt.min for the second subject. The study, thus, demonstrated susceptibility of CP and invariance of AWC to hypoxia. Nevertheless, the study has been conducted with only two subjects in rather severe hypoxia (equivalent to exposure to about 20-22,000 ft) and more importantly, subjects seem to have recovered in hypoxia between two exercise bouts. Additionally, the duration of exposure to hypoxia before CP testing is also not mentioned in the study. It is to be appreciated that both duration of initial exposure to hypoxia (before CP testing) and a hypoxic environment during recovery are likely to affect the test outcome. Severe hypoxia can be hypothesised to impede ATP and PCr homeostasis and thus affect AWC (Roach & Kayser, 2001).

Present study examined robustness of the CP testing protocol during exposure to acute hypobaric hypoxia (equivalent to exposure to 6,000 ft and 10,000 ft) simulated in an altitude chamber. Since an intent was on the examination of the theoretical validity of the concept (and not the performance, *per se*), subjects were made to recover in normoxia between two exercise efforts (*vide infra* in methods). It was hypothesized that even mild hypoxic exposure (equivalent to exposure to 6,000 ft and 10,000 ft) will affect CP but not the AWC.

METHODS

The experimentation was a repeated measure (within subject) evaluation of 14 male nonsmokers who volunteered to participate in the study. The nature and purpose of the study and the risk involved were explained to these volunteers who were ascertained to be healthy by history, physical examination and resting ECG. Subjects were largely sedentary with no significant history of endurance training in the last one year. The protocol was approved by the **Institutes' Ethical Committee**. A written consent was obtained. Physical attributes of the subjects are as follows, age: 30 ± 1 yr, height- 169 ± 1 cm and weight- 68 ± 2 kg (values are mean $\pm$ SE).

All the experimentation was carried out in the hypobaric chamber available in the Department of High Altitude Physiology at the Institute of Aerospace Medicine (IAF), Bangalore situated at an elevation of approximately 963 meters (3,159') from the mean sea level. Dry and wet bulb readings in the chamber varied between 22-27°C and 19-24°C, respectively. Each subject participated in four sessions on different days separated from each other by a period of at least three days.

In the first session, subjects underwent incremental exercise protocol on a cycle ergometer (Corival from Lode, Groningen, The Netherlands) for the measurement of PWC170 i.e., workload which elicited a heart rate of 170 beats per minute. The height of the seat was adjusted to ensure about 15° knee joint angle at full leg extension. Subjects pedaled at the rate of 70 rpm. Starting with a load of 100 watts, exercise continued for three stages with load increasing by 25 watts every four minutes. Heart rate was continuously monitored and last two readings in the last 15 s of each minute of exercise were recorded. Average of the last two readings at the fourth min was taken for each work load. Heart rate value for each work rate was plotted against corresponding work rate and the PWC170 was regressed as the workload corresponding to a heart rate of 170 bpm.

The second to fourth sessions involved determination of CP and AWC using the technique described by Moritani et al (1981). Four dynamic work tests, up to the onset of muscular fatigue were performed on the cycle ergometer in the maximum time or T_{Limit} beyond which the initial power output levels could no longer be maintained i.e., when there was a drop in pedaling frequency below 30 rotations per min (rpm). This ergometer is a constant power device, so that such a drop in rpm results in torque increase which brings about a sharp and well defined end point to an exercise bout. The power output levels were kept sufficiently high (200, 225, 250 and 275 watts) to lead to the onset of muscular fatigue. Rest period was provided between tests for a period of 30 minutes or longer if necessary for heart rate to return within ± 5 bpm of the resting value. The total amount of work performed (W_{Limit}) was defined as the product of the imposed power loading P and the T_{Limit} (i.e., $W_{Limit} = P. T_{Limit}$). CP and AWC were derived as slope coefficient (b) and Y-intercept (a), respectively, of the line defined by the relationship between W_{Limit} and T_{Limit}. (See Fig. 1).

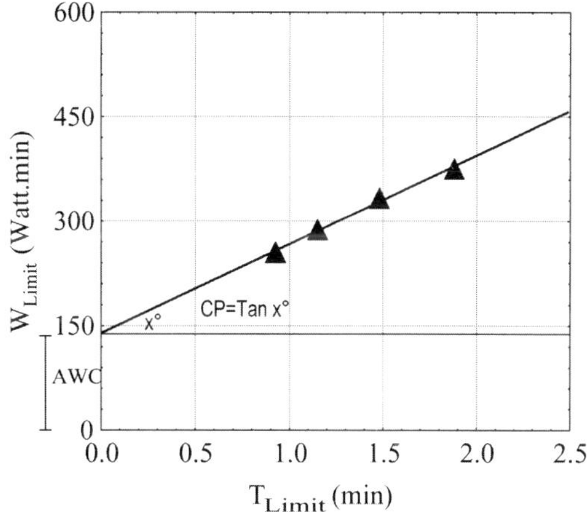

Fig. 1 The figure shows linear relationship between W_{Limit} and T_{Limit} and derivation of CP & AWC as slope coefficient (b) and Y-intercept (a), respectively of the line

CP and AWC measurements, in the second session, were made at ground level (3,159′) with the doors of the chamber closed in order to keep the thermal ambience comparable with that during 'high altitude' evaluations. In the third and the fourth session, chamber was decompressed to simulated altitudes of 6,000 ft and 10,000 ft, respectively. Measurements were made immediately after ascent. After the exercise, a 'descent' was executed to ground level. Therefore, between any two work bouts, subjects recovered in normoxia. Rate of 'ascent' and descent' was kept constant at 3,000 ft per minute for both the altitude simulations. A separate ear clearance run was not done.

Since there is evidence of a circadian rhythm in aerobic and anaerobic responses to high intensity short duration exercise (Hill et al. 1992; Marth et al. 1998), all the experimentation was done in the late afternoons.

Subjects were monitored continuously for Hb saturation and ECG in Standard Lead-II configuration using an Agilent (M 3046 A) Monitor.

Statistics

All the values are presented as mean ± SE (Standard Error). Normality of distribution was examined using Shapiro-Wilk's 'W' statistic. Mauchley's test was used to examine sphericity. A repeated measure (within subject) Analysis of Variance (ANOVA) was used for group comparisons. After a significant outcome from ANOVA, individual comparisons were made using Least Significance Difference (LSD) test. On account of multiple CP values (n = 14) at a given altitudes, regression with replication was (and not with the mean values at each altitude) used as suggested by Zar (2003).

RESULTS

Table 1 and Fig. 2 refer.

Table 1 Physical work capacity (pwc$_{170}$), critical power and anaerobic work capacity at ground level and at the two altitudes

	Ground Level	6,000 ft	10,000 ft	Comparisons*
	[1]	[2]	[3]	
PWC$_{170}$ (watts)	141 ± 6	—	—	—
CP (watts)	136 ± 5	115 ± 8	96 ± 7	F = 13.5; p = 0.000 1 vs 2; p = 0.011 1 vs 3; p = 0.000 2 vs 3; p = 0.021
CP (% of PWC$_{170}$ GL)	98 ± 4	81 ± 4	68 ± 4	F = 13.1; p = 0.000 1 vs 2; p = 0.009 1 vs 3; p = 0.000 2 vs 3; p = 0.032
AWC (watt.min)	133 ± 10	147 ± 14	150 ± 14	F = 0.98; p = 0.388
r$_2$	0.974 ± 0.006	0.978 ± 0.006	0.973 ± 0.005	—

Note: In the column 'comparisons', overall significance of comparison and value of 'F' statistic are followed by outcome of individual comparisons using Least Significant Difference Test.

r$_2$ is the goodness of fit between T$_{Limit}$ and W$_{Limit}$ It is to be appreciated that values larger than 0.774 & 0.921 indicate a significantly linear relationship at p < 0.05 & p < 0.01 levels, respectively.

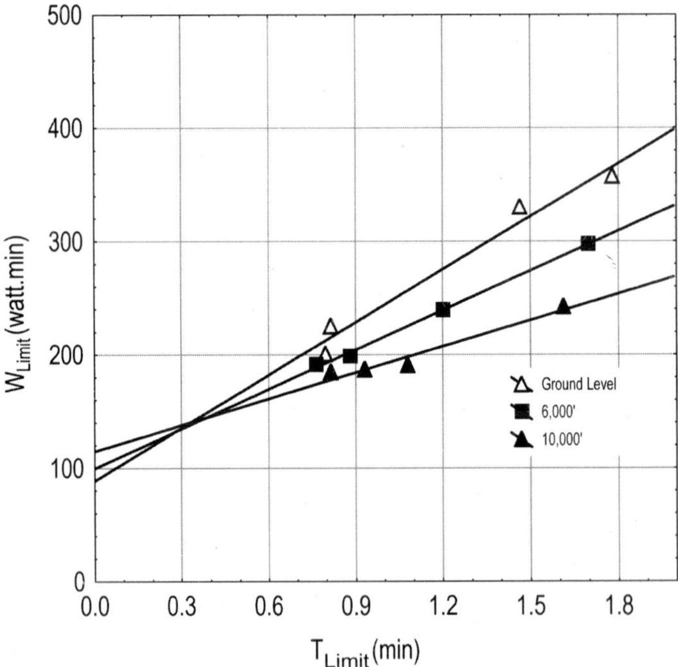

Fig. 2 Effect of acute hypobaric hypoxia on intercept and slope relationship between W$_{Limit}$ & T$_{Limit}$ drawn from the data of a representative subject. It can be seen that hypoxia had a significant effect on the slope, and not on the intercept of the linear regression of W$_{Limit}$ on T$_{Limit}$.

CP decreased significantly from its ground level value of 136 ± 5 watts, to 115 ± 8 watts at 6,000' and 96 ± 7 watts at 10,000' (F = 13.5; p = 0.000). The above change represented a reduction of about 15 ± 5% at 6,000' and 28 ± 6% at 10,000'. CP accounted for 98 ± 4% of PWC_{170} at ground level. This value declined significantly (F = 13.1; p = 0.000) to 81 ± 4% and 68 ± 4% at 6,000' and 10,000', respectively.

On the other hand, no significant effect of altitude was noticed on anaerobic work capacity (F = 0.98; p = 0.388). The values attained by AWC were 133 ± 10, 147 ± 14 and 150 ± 14 watt.min at ground level, 6,000 ft and 10,000 ft, respectively. It is remarkably apparent from Figure 2 that hypoxia affected only the slope and not the intercept of the linear regression of W_{limit} on T_{Limit}.

DISCUSSION

The present study examined the effects of acute hypobaric hypoxia on the outcome of CP testing procedure. Both CP and AWC were evaluated at ground level (at Bangalore situated at approximately 963 m or 3,159 ft above mean sea level) and two altitudes (6,000 ft and 10,000 ft) simulated in a hypobaric chamber. Subjects performed four dynamic work tests (200, 225, 250 and 275 watts) on a cycle ergometer in the maximum time or TLimit and recovered in normoxia between two exercise efforts.

EFFECT OF ACUTE HYPOBARIC HYPOXIA ON CP

Normoxic (ground level) value of CP was 136 ± 5 watts. Earlier, Tripathi & Banerjee (2000) has reported a comparable value of 124±8 watts in a group of 12 untrained subjects with physical attributes comparable to those for the subjects in the present study. As expected, CP decreased significantly during exposure to hypobaric hypoxia (representing a reduction of about 15 ± 5% at 6,000 ft and 28 ± 6% at 10,000 ft). We could not find any systematic study which examined CP on a reasonable number of subject, in a hypoxic ambience comparable to that employed in the present study. In their singular study, Moritani et al (1981), evaluated CP in two subjects who were rendered hypoxic with a gas mixture (with 9% oxygen, equivalent to exposure to 20-22,000 ft altitude). In the two subjects, CP decreased from its normoxic value of 197 watts and 230 watts (while breathing 20.93% oxygen) to 110 watts and 102 (while breathing 9.0% oxygen). It represented a reduction of about 44% and 65% in the two subjects, respectively.

Nonetheless, a reduction in AT, a variable considered analogous to CP, of about 16% is reported by Koistinen et al (1995) in a group of 12 athletes at 3,000 m simulated altitude. These figures are for oxygen uptake (ml/kg/min) at AT determined from ventilatory parameters. Expressing in terms of oxygen uptake as l/min at AT, a reduction of 13% and 28% (derived from blood lactate and ventilatory parameters, respectively) is seen from the results of Ozcelik et al (2004) who simulated hypoxia with a gas mixture of 12% oxygen. Reduction in AT reported in these two studies is apparently much less compared to that observed in the present study for comparable hypoxia. This variance is because AT, in these studies is expressed in terms of oxygen uptake (and not in watts). Such a representation attenuates the changes due to an overall reduction in physical work capacity during hypoxia.

The above noted decrease in CP during exposure to acute hypobaric hypoxia was linear in the altitude range studied in the present study. CP could be regressed from altitude with the following equation (Fig. 3 refers):

$$CP = 137.8 - 3.9. \text{ altitude in 1,000 ft}$$

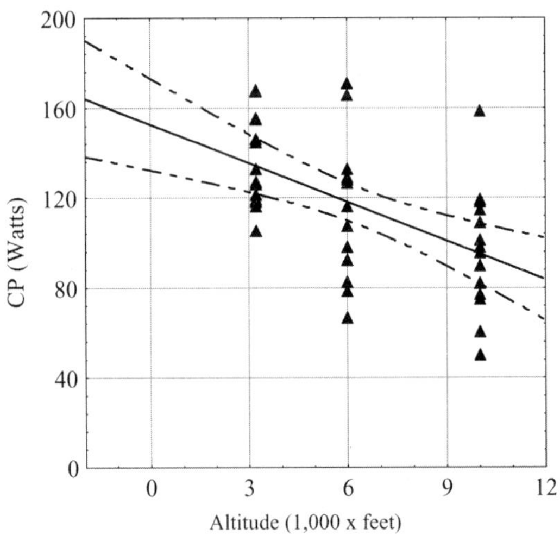

Fig. 3 Effect of acute hypobaric hypoxia on CP. A linear relation was seen with following regression equation–
CP (in watts) = 137 – 4 × altitude (in 1,000 ft)
(F = 15.75, p < 0.0003 & SE of estimate = 2.42)
The two dotted lines indicate 95% confidence limits.

In the above regression, a small error variance indicates a fair prediction of CP.

Nonetheless normoxic values of CP were as high as PWC_{170} and thus appeared to be the maximal power loading which could be maintained for a long duration of time without exhaustion. The observation is apparently at variance with the CP theory and findings of certain studies (Moritani et al. 1981) reporting statistically comparable values of CP and AT with a strong correlation between the two. However, it is to be appreciated that a statistically significant invariance and/or correlation do not establish that two data are in agreement with each other. For a review, please refer to (Bland & Altman, 1986). There are studies which do suggest that CP overestimates the power that can be maintained continuously. Housh et al (1989) found that eleven out of fourteen of their subjects could not maintain exercise on cycle ergometer at their estimated CP for one hour. Average endurance was found to be 33.31 minutes. They also observed that CP represented a power loading which was approximately 17% greater than that which could be maintained for 60 minutes. Jenkins & Quigley (1990) found six out of eight cyclist and McLellan & Cheung [1992] found 13 out of 14 subjects unable to maintain CP for 30 min without exhaustion. In the former study (Jenkins & Quigley, 1990), the mean power attained over 30 minutes was 6.4% below their estimated CP. A very similar conclusion has been drawn by Pepper et al (1992) for treadmill running at critical velocity. Average time to exhaustion at estimated CP was found to be even lower, at only 16.43 min. In an earlier study, Tripathi & Banerjee (2000) found CP to be 26%, 24% and 23% higher than AT, both having been expressed in watts, VO_2 (l/min) and VO2 (ml/kg/min), respectively. In the present study, normoxic values of CP were almost comparable to PWC_{170}.

A positive bias in the estimation of CP (and a negative bias in the estimation of AWC) is hypothesised by Vandewalle et al. (1989) due to time lag in oxygen delivery (against the assumption of immediate availability of the CP component even in CP theory), the fact that oxygen delivery takes time to reach a steady.

EFFECT OF ACUTE HYPOBARIC HYPOXIA ON AWC

No significant effect of altitude was noticed on anaerobic work capacity. The values attained by AWC were 133 ± 10, 147 ± 14 and 150 ± 14 watt.min at ground level, 6,000' and 10,000', respectively. The normoxic values are statistically comparable to those observed by the author (155 ± 10 watt.min) in studies on untrained volunteers evaluated at ground level at Bangalore (Tripathi & Banerjee 2000). Moritani et al (1981) have reported significantly higher values in his study of 16 college students (8 male and 8 female subjects). AWC values for the male and female subjects were 226.5 ± 63.4 watt.min and 143.6 ± 12.6 watt.min, respectively. However, subjects in their study were significantly younger and more fit physically (as is suggested from the values of maximal oxygen uptake). It is quite possible that their subjects were different in terms of anthropometric attributes as well (physical attributes other than age are not given by the authors in the article). Notwithstanding the above variation and its explanation, a remarkable observation in all these studies is a wide individual variation as appears from high values of SE and large confidence intervals. A pronounced individual variability is also apparent from the data of McLellan & Cheung (1992), re-analysed by Morton (1996). AWC in this study is reported to be 16836 ± 1255 joules.

A pertinent question arises as to why an effect was not seen in AWC of hypoxia which is reported to increase anaerobic metabolism. There could be following reasons for this: **1)** such a phenomenon is observed only at the onset of square-wave exercise when an energy deficit (due to slowed O_2 uptake-on response) is to be made good, transiently. This inference is largely based on the observations that performance during explosive efforts (not exceeding 30-45 sec) is unaffected under hypoxia despite an apparent reduction in O_2 uptake which is accompanied by a significantly larger lactate accumulation. In contradistinction to such short explosive efforts, during maximal exhaustive exercise (which is used in CP testing) the end point of subjective fatigue is largely decided by blood lactate levels which are not different in acute hypoxia from those in normoxia (Lundby et al, 2000). As a matter of fact, hypoxia is shown not to have any effect on the amplitude of the primary rise in oxygen uptake (period of first 2–3 min of exercise). In view of the above synthesis, it is reasonable to conceive that AWC, as measured from CP testing protocol will be accommodative of slowing of O_2 uptake-on response at the onset of exercise. Linnarsson et al (1974) observed that oxygen deficit, muscle ATP, muscle creatine phosphate (CP) and muscle or blood lactate concentrations were not different significantly after maximal exercise in acute hypobaric hypoxia (0.68 ATA simulated in a decompression chamber) did not result significantly from the corresponding values when the exercise was performed in normoxia (1 ATA). This was despite a significant reduction in the performance time and maximal oxygen uptake during hypoxia. It is also noteworthy that a number of studies have failed to find any reduction in O_2 uptake-on response during exposure to such a mild hypoxia as simulated in the present study (Griffiths et al, 1986).

IMPRESSION WITH REFERENCE TO CP THEORY

A decrease in CP with altitude hypoxia supports its aerobic derivation, at least partially. There are three main mechanisms (Calbet et al, 2003) which account for the reduction of aerobic capacity in acute hypoxia: **1)** reduction of inspired oxygen tension, **2)** impairment of pulmonary gas exchange and **3)** reduction of maximal cardiac output. Each of these mechanisms are shown to contribute to about one-third of the loss in maximal aerobic power. Nonetheless, decrease in CP during hypoxia seems to be attenuated die to increasing contribution from anaerobic mechanisms which tend to increase transiently during such exposures. Similarly, an invariance of AWC during exposure to mild hypoxia submits an indirect validation to the theory of CP testing procedure. Additionally, we were conscious to the fact that an apparently linear relation between W_{Limit} and T_{Limit} may be due to a statistical 'illusion'. It can be shown that if there are only two data points, correlation will always be perfect (r will always be 1.00). With three data points and only one degree of freedom left (as is usually done during CP testing protocol), values larger than 0.95 and 0.99 will only be significant at $p < 0.05$ and $p < 0.01$ levels, respectively. The corresponding values for four data points would be 0.88 and 0.96. Due to these reasons, we calculated the individual values of r_2. It seems that the concept holds good as is apparent from the values of r_2.

CONCLUSION

To the best of our appreciation, this is the first systemic study which employed hypobaric hypoxia to examine the validity of CP testing procedure with a reasonable number of subjects. The uniqueness of the study is that subjects recovered in normoxia between any two exercise bouts. Our results endorse the theoretical validity of the concept. Nevertheless, CP component appeared to be closer to PWC_{170} with some contribution from anaerobic mechanisms.

REFERENCES

Bland JM, Altman DG (1986) Statistical methods for assessing agreement between two methods of clinical measurement. Lancet i: 307-310

Calbet JAL, Boushel R, Rådegran G, Søndergaard H, Wagner PD, Saltin B (2003) Determinants of maximal oxygen uptake in severe acute hypoxia. Am J Physiol Regul Integr Comp Physiol 284: 291-303

deVries HA, Tichy MW, Housh TJ, Smyth KD, Tichy AM, Housh DJ (1987) A method for estimating physical working capacity at the fatigue threshold (PWCFT). Ergonomics 30:1195-1204

Engelen M, Porszasz J, Riley M, Wasserman K, Maehara K, Barstow TJ (1996) Effects of hypoxic hypoxia on O2 uptake and heart rate kinetics during heavy exercise. J Appl Physiol81: 2500-2508

Gaesser GA, Wilson LA (1988) Effects of continuous and interval training on the parameters of the power-endurance time relationship for high-intensity exercise. Int J Sports Med 9: 417-421

Griffiths TL, Henson LC, Whipp BJ (1986) Influence of inspired oxygen concentration on the dynamics of the exercise hyperpnoea in man. J Physiol 380: 387-403

Hill DW, Borden DO, Darnaby KM, Hendricks DN, Hill CM (1992) Effect of time of day on aerobic and anaerobic responses to high-intensity exercise. Can J Sport Sci 17: 316-319

Hill DW, Smith JC (1993). A comparison of methods of estimating anaerobic work capacity. Ergonomics 36: 1495-1500

Housh DJ, Housh TJ, Bauge SM (1989) The accuracy of the critical power test for predicting time to exhaustion during cycle ergometry. Ergonomics 32: 997-1004

Jenkins DG, Quigley BM (1990) Blood lactate in trained cyclists during cycle ergometry at critical power. Eur J Appl Physiol Occup Physiol 61: 278-283

Jenkins DG, Quigley BM (1991) The y-intercept of the critical power function as a measure of anaerobic work capacity. Ergonomics 34: 13-22

Jenkins DG, Quigley BM (1992) Endurance training enhances critical power. Med Sci Sports Exerc 24: 1283-1289

Jenkins DG, Quigley BM (1993) The influence of high-intensity exercise training on the Wlim-Tlim relationship. Med Sci Sports Exerc 25: 275-282

Koistinen P, Takala T, Martikkala V, Leppaluoto J (1995) Aerobic fitness influences the response of maximal oxygen uptake and lactate threshold in acute hypobaric hypoxia. Int J Sports Med 16: 78-81

Linnarsson D, Karlsson J, Fagraeus L, Saltin B (1974) Muscle metabolites and oxygen deficit with exercise in hypoxia and hyperoxia. J Appl Physiol 36: 399-402

Lundby C, Saltin B, van Hall G (2000) The 'lactate paradox', evidence for a transient change in the course of acclimatization to severe hypoxia in lowlanders. Acta Physiol Scand 170: 265-269

McLellan TM, Cheung KS (1992) A comparative evaluation of the individual anaerobic threshold and the critical power. Med Sci Sports Exerc 24: 543-550

Marth PD, Woods RR, Hill DW (1998) Influence of time of day on anaerobic capacity. Percept Mot Skills 86: 592-594

Miura A, Kino F, Kajitani S, Sato H, Fukuba Y (1999) The effect of oral creatine supplementation on the curvature constant parameter of the power-duration curve for cycle ergometry in humans. Jpn J Physiol 49: 169-74

Monod H, Scherrer J (1965) The work capacity of a synergic muscular group. Ergonomics 8:329-338

Moritani T, Nagata A, deVries HA, Muro M (1981) Critical power as a measure of physical work capacity and anaerobic threshold. Ergonomics 24: 339-50

Morton RH (1996) A 3-parameter critical power model. Ergonomics 39: 611-619.

Ozcelik O, Kelestimur H (2004) Effects of acute hypoxia on the determination of anaerobic threshold using the heart rate-work rate relationships during incremental exercise tests. Physiol Res 53: 45-51

Pepper ML, Housh TJ, Johnson GO (1992) The accuracy of the critical velocity test for predicting time to exhaustion during treadmill running. Int J Sports Med 13: 121-124

Roach R, Kayser B (2001) Exercise and hypoxia. In: Hornbein TF, Schoene RB (eds). High Altitude, An exploration of human adaptation. Marcel Dekker, Inc New York, pp 663-705

Smith JC, Stephens DP, Hall EL, Jackson AW, Earnest CP (1998) Effect of oral creatine ingestion on parameters of the work rate time relationship and time to exhaustion in highintensity cycling. Eur J Appl Physiol 77:360–365

Stout JR, Eckerson JM, JHT, Ebersole KT (1999) The effects of creatine supplementation on anaerobic working capacity. J Strength Cond Res 13: 135–138

Tripathi KK, Banerjee PK (2000) A comparative evaluation of critical power and anaerobic threshold as determinants of work intensity that can be maintained without the onset of metabolic fatigue. In: Majumdar D & Selvamurthy W (eds), Advances in Ergonomics, Occupational Health and Safety. New Age International (P) Limited, New Delhi, pp 122-128

Vandewalle H, Kapitaniak B, Grun S, Raveneau S, Monod H (1989) Comparison between a 30-s all-out test and a time-work test on a cycle ergometer Eur J Appl Physiol Occup Physiol 58: 375-381

Weyand PG, Lee CS, Martinez-Ruiz R, Bundle MW, Bellizzi MJ, Wright S (1999) Highspeed running performance is largely unaffected by hypoxic reductions in aerobic power. J Appl Physiol 86: 2059-2064

Zar JH (2003) Simple linear regression. In: Biostatistical Analysis.Pearson Education Inc., Delhi, pp 324-359

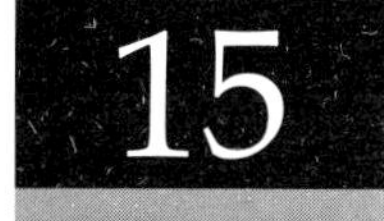

Muscular Strength Changes in Women aged 45-50 years following Resistance Training

Usha S. Nair and Leena Christie

LNCPE, Sports Authority of India, Trivandrum

ABSRACT

The purpose of this study was to determine the muscular strength changes in women who undertook six weeks of resistance training. The subjects were forty women selected at random (n = 20) experimental and (n = 20) control group between the age group of 45 – 50 years from Trivandrum. Strength was assessed by 1 RM. Muscular strength test was done for biceps curl, shoulder press, chest press, lateral pull down and leg curl. The 1 RM assessment was done before and after six weeks of resistance training. The experimental group underwent six weeks of resistance training. Results: t-test values for the experimental group for each of the strength tests for groups for biceps curl, shoulder press, chest press, lateral pull down and leg curl were12.85, 8.10, 14.03, 11.8 and 9.59 respectively. While the t-values were not significant for the control group. Even though strength declines with aging, the results of the study indicated 6 weeks of resistance training can result in improvement of strength in biceps curl, shoulder press, chest press, lateral pull down and leg curl in women aged 45–50 years of age.

INTRODUCTION

Midlife can be a time when life challenges come from many directions. Falling levels of estrogen and progesterone are associated with changes in muscle recovery fat deposition, mental function, and joint discomfort, sleep disturbances and dry skin.

The loss of estrogen associated with menopause is related to high level of autoimmune and inflammatory disorders in midlife and older women. The condition such as shoulder bursitis and fibromyalagia are not uncommon. The shoulders of women are susceptible because of change in spinal alignment and stress to shoulder during child bearing. Strength in hips and legs are important in maintaining maximum balance range and coordinated stability.

Age is a major determinant of bone strength, mass and microarchitecture as well as muscle mass. These factors are also affected by loading. By the time the women is perimenopausal she is losing bone and muscle mass. One study indicates that there is concomitant loss of muscle strength and bone density in women between 45 and 65 years irrespective of HRT, and that the loss of lower body strength is 50 % greater than the loss of upper body strength.

Women are especially at risk after menopause when the bone protective effects of estrogen are lost. At one time loss of function in the elderly was attributed to the aging process. That belief is now being challenged as studies show gain in physiological performance with exercise in older persons.

Women can have their peak bone mineral density (BMD) in their teens or twenties, maintain their bone mass in their thirties, but in their forties it is critical that women are doing activities that load bone especially the spine, pelvis and the femur to help minimize bone and muscle loss.

Snow et al (2000) found that the exercise programme helps prevent significant loss of femoral neck, trochanter and total hip BMD in older postmenopausal women.

Strength training is an effective means to reduce the risk and manage many conditions associated with aging. Strength loss contributes to osteoporotic decline in bone density and arthritis joint pain. Strength rather than cardiovascular function is considered to be the most physiologically limiting factor for the elderly (Coleman et al, 1996). Many elderly persons become dependent after only a mild illness due to minimal physiologic reserves (Lancet, 1986).

Sarcopenia is the name given to age related muscle mass decline (Butler, 1993) muscle strength declines 5% per decade after the age of 45 (Aoyagi and Shepherd, 1992) and 15%per decade after age 60 (Taunton et al, 1997) A declining number of fibers and denervation of fibers are the key causes of loss of muscular force in older persons (Coleman et al, 1996). Gill's study (1995) identifies that the pattern of independence loss begins with the functional tasks which are more dependent on lower extremity and trunk performance. The magnitude of strength gain with older adult varies depending on the subjects' initial functional level, training programme, and exercise intensity. Perkins & Kaiser (1961) found 57% strength gains following six weeks of isotonic strength training in persons over 60. In a 24 weeks study, Nicholas et al, achieved strength gains ranging from 5% - 65% with elderly women. Fiatarone et al (1994) found 11.3% strength increase in 10-week strength training study of frail elderly.

The purpose of this investigation was to examine muscular strength changes in biceps curl, shoulder press, chest press, lateral pull down and leg curl following six weeks of resistance training on midlife women.

METHODOLOGY

Participants

Participants selected were females aged 45 to 50 years from Trivandrum who were not taking any hormone or such medication. All the women had not participated in any structured exercise programme. Subject chosen for the study received medical clearance to begin resistance exercise training programme. Subject's recruitment was done through community centres. All the participants gave their written informed consent to participate.

Procedure

The subjects were randomly assigned to an experimental group (n = 20) and control group (n = 20). Muscular strength was assessed by one repetition maximum testing (1 RM). Lateral pull down, leg curl, chest press and shoulder press was done on plate loaded exercise machines. Biceps curl was done with smaller rods and plates. All the test was done in the following sequence: lateral pull down, chest press, leg press, shoulder press and biceps curl. Each test began with a general warm up and five repetition of each exercise with 3 minutes rest. A single repetition was then attempted with a heavier weight followed by 4 minutes rest. This sequence was repeated until the subject's 1RM were achieved. 1 RM strength was assessed at the baseline and after six weeks of training period for both the experimental and control group.

The lateral pull down was done from a seated position with the bar being pulled to chin level in front of the head. The chest press was done on a horizontal bench, starting with the arms parallel to the floor. In the leg curl the seat was positioned to place the participants' knees at 90 degrees angle when in starting position. The shoulder press was done flexed arms parallel to the floor. Biceps curl was done in standing position with both the arms.

Training Protocol

The training period consisted of six weeks supervised exercise programme. Participants exercised thrice a week with a minimum of 48 hours rest between sessions. The exercise programme consisted of five resistance exercises; biceps curl, shoulder press, chest press, leg curl and lateral pull down. The participants performed two sets of 12 -15 repetition, preceded by a 10 minutes warm up followed by stretching. Plate loaded equipment was used for exercise session. The initial training load by percentage of 1 RM. The participants recorded their weights used and repetition completed on exercise log during each session. An increase in resistance occurred once 15 repetitions were completed successfully.

Statistical Analysis

The statistical method used was a comparison of two means using a paired t test. The level of significance was set at p < 0.05.

RESULTS

The results of the first weeks are presented in Table 1. Significant improvement in muscle strength was seen in biceps curl, shoulder press, chest press, chest press, leg curl and lateral pull down in the exercising group. The control group had no significant changes in the muscle strength for any of the exercise.

Table 1 Six weeks changes in weight exercisers.

Group	Lateral Pull down	Chest press	Leg curl	Shoulder press	Biceps curl
Experimental Mean (kg)					
Baseline	24.15	10.60	18.85	12.20	5.0
After 6 weeks	28.45	12.90	22.85	14.90	7.5
SD (kg) Baseline	5.83	4.27	4.17	3.19	2.96
After 6 weeks	5.36	4.18	4.13	4.18	3.01
n	20	20	20	20	20
t value	11.18	14.03	9.59	8.10	12.85
Significant Improvement at 1 %	yes	yes	yes	yes	yes
Control Mean (kg)					
Baseline	18.80	10.60	15.9	12.40	5.0
After 6 weeks SD (kg)	18.70	10.50	16.05	12.30	5.10
Baseline	3.77	2.19	3.02	2.10	2.27
After 6 weeks	3.64	2.07	3.01	1.90	2.29
n	20	20	20	20	20
t value	1.0	1.0	1.37	.80	.70
Significant Improvementat 5%	no	no	no	no	no

DISCUSSION

Significant improvement was seen in all the selected muscle strength variables in the exercising group. It may probably be due to the fact that women experience similar strength gains compared to men who participated in the strength training programmes, but they do not experience similar hypertrophy. The increase in strength may be due to neural control of trained muscle, which is altered, allowing greater force production (Donag et al, 1984).

The subjects in this study were sedentary, could have resulted in significant improvement, as the initial level of fitness was low. The subjects following the training felt very energetic and those activities, which were previously considered impossible, were now possible. This psychosocial change may lead to increased levels of activities, which could help to prolong independence. They could carry themselves in a better way.

CONCLUSION

This study has shown that six weeks of resistance training has resulted in improvement of strength in biceps curl, shoulder press, chest press, lateral pull down and leg curl in women 45 -50 years of aged women.

References

1. Humphries, B., Triplett Mc Bride, T., Newton, R.U., Marshal, S. 1999. The relationship between dynamic isokinetic and isometric strength and bone mineral density in a population of 45 to 65 years old women. Journal of science and medicine in sport 2 94): 367-374

2. Coleman E. A., Buchner, D.M., Cress M.E., Chan B.K., Delateur B.J. The relationship of joint symptoms with exercise performance in older adults. Journal of American geriatrics society, 44: 14-21, 1996

3. Snow, C.M., Shaw, J.M., Winters, K.M. and Witske, K.A. Long term exercise using weighted vests prevents hip bone loss in postmenopausal women. The journal of gerontology, Biological science and medical science. 55 (9): M489-491.

4. Fiatarone, M.A., Neil, E.F., Ryan, N.D., Clememts, K.M., Solares, G.R., Nelson, M.E. Exercise training and nutritional supplementation for physical frailty in very elderly people. New England journal of medicine. 330: 1769-1773, 1994.

5. Tiidus, P.M 1999. Nutritional implications of gender differences in metabolism, estrogen and oxygen radicals, oxidative damage, inflammation and muscle function. In Tarnopolsky (ed), Gender differences in metabolism. Baton Raton, FL; CRC Press

6. Buchner, D.M. and Wagner, E.H. Preventive frail health. Clinical geriatricmedicine. 8: 1-17, 1992.

7. Butler, R.N. Did you say 'sarcopenia'? Geriatrics. 48: 11-12, 1993.

8. Aoyagi y. and Shepherd, R.J. Aging and muscle function. Sports medicine, 14(6): 376-396. 1992.

9. Gill, T.M., Williams, M.E. Assessing risk for the onset of functional dependence among older adults: The role of physical performance. Journal of American Geriatric society, 43: 603-609, 1995.

10. The Lancet. Physical activity in old age. 1431, 1986.

11. Taunton, J.E., Martin, E.C., r hodes, L.A., wolski, Elliot, J. Exercise for older woman: choosing the right prescription, British journal of sports medicine, 31: 5-10, 1997

12. Perkins, L.C., Kaiser, H.L. Results of short term isotonic and isometric exercise programme in persons over sixty. Physical therapy review, 41: 633-635, 1961.

16

Hydration in Sportspersons

G.L. Khanna

Dean (Academics) Department of Therapies and Health Sciences
Faridabad Institute of Technology
Manav Rachna Educational Institutions
Faridabad

ABSTRACT

Loss of fluid electrolyte and reduction of the body's carbohydrate stores are the major causes of fatigue in prolonged exhaustive exercise. Dehydration resulting from sweat loss, and increase in core temperature may be primary cause of fatigue Though sweat loss in high intensity, short duration exercise is small, exercise capacity is impaired if there is a pre-exercise fluid deficit. Fluid ingestion during exercise has the twin benefits of providing a source of carbohydrate fluid to supplement the body's limited store, and of supplying water to replace losses caused by sweating. Several studies have indicated that carbohydrate supplementation during prolonged exercise improves endurance performance by maintaining blood glucose level. Electrolyte content of the fluid maintains the electrolyte balance and reduces the onset of fatigue. Effect of electrolyte and water replacement on cardiovascular system endurance and recovery will be discussed.

INTRODUCTION

Loss of fluid electrolyte and reduction of the body's carbohydrate stores are the major causes of fatigue in prolonged exhaustive exercise (Wilmore and Costill, 2004, Maughan et al., 2007;). Dehydration resulting from sweat loss, and increase in core temperature may be primary cause of fatigue (Maughan et al., 2007; Wilmore and Costill, 2004). Electrolyte content of the fluid maintains the electrolyte balance and reduces the onset of fatigue (Byrne et al., 2005; Khanna and Manna, 2005). It is reported that sweat loss in high intensity, short duration exercise is small, exercise capacity is impaired if there is a pre-exercise fluid deficit. Fluid ingestion during exercise has the twin benefits of providing a source of carbohydrate fluid to supplement the body's limited store, and of supplying water to replace losses caused by sweating (McArdle et al. 2001; Wilmore and Costill, 2004). Several studies have indicated that carbohydrate supplementation during prolonged exercise improves endurance performance by maintaining blood glucose level (Byrne et al., 2005; Shirreffs et al., 2007).

Water in the body is distributed between two compartments, the intracellular fluid (ICF) - water inside cells and extracellular fluid (ECF) - water outside cells (Guyton and Hall, 2000 The main factors responsible for the regulation of water balance are fluid volume and osmolarity . there is no net movement of water between the ICF and the ECF if the ECF osmolarity is normal. If the osmolarity of the ECF increases and becomes hypertonic relative to the cells then water diffuses from the cells into the ECF (Guyton and Hall, 2000). Sweat is hypotonic in relation to blood, dehydration from exercise causes an increase in serum osmolarity (McArdle et al. 2001; Wilmore and Costill, 2004). Both hypovolemia and hyperosmolarity increase internal temperature and reduce heat dissipation from evaporation and convection. Serum hyperosmolarity may increase internal temperature, affecting the hypothalamus and/or sweat glands, delaying the starting of sweat and peripheral vasodilation during exercise (McArdle et al. 2001; Wilmore and Costill, 2004).

It has been reported by several scientists that with 1 to 2% dehydration, body temperature starts rising in up to 0.4oC for each subsequent dehydration, between 4 to 6%, thermal fatigue may occur; from 6% on, there is the risk of thermal shock, coma and death. Greater losses of 4% can reduce high-intensity exercise capacity (eg maximal cycling) by up to 50% due to a reduced VO2max, while reducing skeletal muscle performance by 15% (McArdle et al. 2001; Wilmore and Costill, 2004).

EFFECT ON AEROBIC PERFORMANCE

Aerobic performance is significantly affected by loss of water.It is observed that loss of 1L of water via sweating from the circulating blood volume can deteriorate the efficiency of heart and circulation and considerably reduce its performance. Thus major target of fluid replacement during exercise and recovery is to maintain volume. Decrease in plasma volume has been reported to increase in heart rate and stroke volume and also the hearts ability to maintain its out put (Shirreffs and Maughan, 2006).

Athletes has to be hydrated prior to competition, training and exercise. In addition to drinking fluid in the 24 hours before an exercise session, the ACSM has recommended drinking 400 to 600 mL of fluid 2-3 hours before exercise. It improves the hydration status of athletes and does not lead to deterioration of performance in the competition and also have deleterious effect on various physiological systems.

The factors which influence in maintaining plasma volume are:

1. Ability of the ingested solution to transverse the stomach and get absorbed in the intestine.
2. Gastric emptying rates and intestinal absorption may have impact on actual performance.
3. Gastric emptying is facilitated by intake of low-calories fluids, and intestinal absorption is optimized with isosmotic fluids between 200 and 260 mosmol/kg.
4. Intake of hypertonic fluids could cause body water to be secreted to the intestinal lumen.
5. Other factors like taste of the fluid affect temperature, sweetness, intensity of flavor and acidity, sensation of thirst etc

SODIUM REPLACEMENT

Sportsperson may lose two liters of sweat per hour, total loss of sodium is 240 mEq, i.e., 10% of the total extracellular space Na+. Such loss would be irrelevant, were it not for the risk of hyponatremia, a concentration of serum sodium less than 130 mEq l-1, due to a fluid replacement with sodium-free or low-sodium fluids, particularly in lengthy events (Byrne et al., 2005; Montain et al., 2006).

HYPONATREMIA

Hyponatraemia results from an abnormally low concentration of sodium in blood plasma – the normal range being 136-142 mmol per litre. A sustained decrease in plasma sodium concentration disrupts the osmotic balance across the blood-brain barrier, leading to a rapid influx of water into the brain. This, in turn, leads to swelling of the brain, which can progress to confusion, seizure, coma and even death. (Montain et al., 2006).

Various factors can lead to a fall in sodium concentration, including loss of sodium in sweat and decreased sodium intake. But the rapid intake of large quantities of fluids, which effectively dilutes the blood, appears to be the major cause of dangerous reductions. To avoid hyponatremia, it has been recommended by the scientist to include 0.5 and 0.7 g/L sodium during exercise lasting longer than 1 hour because it may enhance palatability and the drive to drink.During a marathon race, it is recommended to drink 100-200ml of fluid every 15-20 minutes along the way. A drink containing sodium may be preferred (Guyton and Hall, 2000).

Carbohydrate-electrolyte drink on endurance time and cardiovascular response during exercise and recovery was conducted by sports Authority of India (Khanna and Manna, 2005). Total time of endurance at 70 per cent VO2 max was found to increase significantly ($P < 0.01$) following a 5 g per cent carbohydrate-electrolyte drink supplement. The increase of total endurance time was noted about 51 per cent when supplied with carbohydrate-

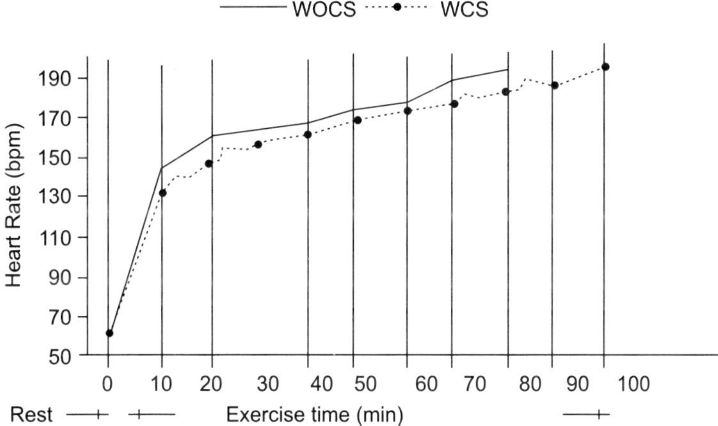

Fig. 1 Heart rate responses during exercise with and without supplementation of carbohydrate-electrolyte drink (n = 10). WOCS, without carbohydrate supplementation; WCS, with carbohydrate supplementation. $P^* < 0.05$; $** < 0.01$; $*** < 0.001$ compared to WOCS.

electrolyte drink. The endurance time recorded with and without carbohydrate-electrolyte drink supplement was 94.1 ± 17.7 and 62.3 ± 10.4 min respectively. Significant improvements in cardiovascular responses were noted during moderate intensity exercise (at 70% VO_{2max}) following a 5 g per cent carbohydrate-electrolyte drink (Fig. 1).

Cardiovascular responses during recovery were also improved significantly after the supplementation of 12.5 g per cent carbohydrate-electrolyte drink (Table II).

Table II Effects of supplementation of 12.5 g% carbohydrate-electrolyte drink on recovery heart rate

Groups	WOCS	WCS
Rec HR1 (bpm)	154 ± 6.1	$148 \pm 6.4*$
Rec HR2 (bpm)	138 ± 6.6	$127 \pm 4.9*$
Rec HR3 (bpm)	118 ± 5.2	$109 \pm 5.8*$

Rec HR1, recovery heart rate after 1st min; Rec HR2, recovery heart rate after 2nd min; Rec HR3, recovery heart rate after 3rd min; WOCS, without carbohydrate supplementation; WCS, with carbohydrate supplementation $*P < 0.05$, $**P < 0.01$

Effect of Carbohydrate-electrolyte Drink on Blood Glucose Levels during Exercise and Recovery

Blood glucose values were noted at rest and then at an interval of 10 min each during exercise and recovery. No significant changes were noted in blood glucose level throughout the exercise period at 70 per cent VO2 max when supplied with 5 g per cent carbohydrate-electrolyte drink. No significant change in blood glucose level was noted during recovery after 10 min (without supplementation 100.8 ± 9.2 mg/dl; with supplementation 108.4 ± 25.6 mg/dl), however, a significantly ($P < 0.01$) higher blood glucose level was noted during recovery after 20 min (without supplementation 100.3 ± 9.9 mg/dl; with supplementation 119.2 ± 10.3 mg/dl) with a 12.5 g per cent carbohydrate-electrolyte drink.

Effect of Carbohydrate-electrolyte Drink on Blood Lactate Levels during Exercise and Recovery

Blood lactate values were noted at rest and then at an interval of 10 min each during exercise and recovery. It was noted that supplementation of 5 g per cent carbohydrate-electrolyte drink keeps the blood lactate at lower levels. Although most of the values were not significant, but significantly lower ($P < 0.01$) value was noted after 70 min of exercise (without supplementation 3.4 ± 0.6 mmol/l compared to 2.1 ± 0.4 mmol/l with supplementation). However, no significant alteration was noted in peak lactate level (without supplementation 3.7 ± 1.2 mmol/l with supplementation 3.2 ± 1.0 mmol/l). Removal of blood lactate was significantly ($P < 0.05$) faster after 10 min (without supplementation 3.1 ± 1.0 mmol/l; with supplementation 2.1 ± 0.8 mmol/l) and 20 min (without supplementation 2.5 ± 0.9 mmol/l; with supplementation 1.5 ± 0.4 mmol/l) with 12.5 g per cent carbohydrate-electrolyte drink. Hypohydration impairs the body's ability to regulate heat resulting in increased body temperature and an elevated heart rate, causing the athlete to feel more fatigued than usual at a given work rate with reduced mental function, followed by slow gastric emptying which results in stomach discomfort. All these effects lead to impairment in exercise performance. There is substantial evidence that consumption of an isotonic sports drink during exercise can improve performance during prolonged sub-maximal, intermittent, high intensity, and shuttle running test (Nicholas et al., 1995). The consumption of isotonic sports drinks either throughout or late in exercise has been shown to delay the onset of tiredness and thus improve performance (Tsintzas et al., 1996a). It may be either due to carbohydrate ingestion preventing a decline in blood glucose and maintaining carbohydrate oxidation at a high rate late in exercise, or due to muscle glycogen sparing early in exercise (Tsintzas et al 1996b; Fallowfield et al., 1995). The amount of pre-exercise muscle glycogen stores is an important factor in determining endurance capacity. Prolonged exercise causes dehydration and reduces the body's carbohydrate energy stores. These are the major contributors to the onset of fatigue. Different mechanisms have been proposed to show that the ergogenic effect of carbohydrate does not affect muscle glycogen at a critical point in endurance exercise when liver and muscle glycogen levels are low and uptake of glycogen by skeletal muscle is increased.

The carbohydrate content of drinks taken should be determined by relative needs to supply fuel and water. This depends on the intensity and duration of the exercise, the ambient temperature and humidity, and on the physiological and biochemical characteristics of the individual athlete. Electrolytes of sodium, magnesium, calcium and potassium help the cells to function normally and provide the key to muscle function, mental focus and body cooling. Electrolytes are easily lost in sweat and urine during physical activity, so replenshing these minerals are important. More severe water loss at high temperatures along with electrolytes puts a person at risk of heat cramps or sometimes heat stroke. Low level of potassium or magnesium enhances muscles cramptor.

In a recently conducted study Coconut water is also found to be as good as ingesting carbohydrate enriched beverages in heat and humidity. In summary, it may be concluded that carbohydrate replacement during exercise may enhance performance of sports and activities, which typically deplete body carbohydrate stores, by providing an additional fuel source for the muscle. Carbohydrate and electrolyte balance keeps low heart rate as well as low blood lactate level during exercise.

Recovery After Exercise

Optimal post-exercise rehydration requires both higher fluid volume replacement and sodium content compared with rehydration during exercise. Ingestion of plain water delays rehydration because it decreases plasma osmolality, reduces thirst and increases freewater clearance. Replacement of sodium lost in sweat is important in maximizing the retention of ingested fluids. Sodium is particularly important for fluid restoration after exercise. The optimum means of replacing fluid and salts lost during exercise is to provide a combination of water, carbohydrate and mineral salts. Water reduces dehydration and helps to maintain blood volume, which improves performance because it lowers the heart rate and body temperature, and mineral salts help to restore electrolyte balance by boosting the process of water absorption.

Muscle glycogen resynthesis is enhanced if carbohydrate beverages are ingested immediately following an exercise bout (Burke et al., 1993). The rate of resynthesis is dependent on the amount of carbohydrate ingested . Ingestion of 50g of glucose and sucrose every 2hour for 6 hours after exercise enhances replenishment and rapid recovery of plasma . The addition of sodium to carbohydrate solutions results in increased replenishment of muscle glycogen (Nielsen et al., 1986).

Recommendations Concerning Fluid Replacement

Natural fruit drinks such as young coconut water has been studied as a post re hydration drink (Saat et.al., 2002). It has a fairly low rehydration index due to high potassium and low sodium content. Later on Che-Ishak (2003) investigated the effectiveness of coconut water by increasing the sodium content up to 20 mmol/l. The sodium enriched coconut water was effective in allowing better restoration of plasma volume and had a good rehydration index. Intake of lemon juice before and after exercise improves performance and delays fatigue. Studies at the University of Memphis exercise and sports nutrition laboratory (2004) found that honey is one of the most effective forms of carbohydrate before, during and after exercise. Recent study conducted by Sports Authority of India has indicated that ingestion of sugar cane juice during and after exercise can enhance performance and recovery (Unpublished data)

One should intake fluids before, during and after practicing exercise. To ensure a good hydration at the beginning of the exercise, it is recommended the drinking of about 250 to 500 ml of water two hours before the exercise. During the exercise, fluid intake should begin within the first 15 minutes, and kept on at every 15 to 20 minutes. The volume to be taken ranges according to sweat rates, from 500 to 2,000 ml/hour. If the activity lasts for more than one hour, or if it is intense, of intermittent type, even lasting less than one hour, one should replace carbohydrate in the amount of 30 to 60 gm/hr and Na+ in the amount of 0.5 to 0.7 gm/lt. The temperature of the beverage should range from 15 to 22°C, and flavored according to individual preference. The beverage should be easy to reach, in bottles that make drinking easy, interrupting the exercise as little as possible. After the exercise, one should keep on drinking fluids to make up for additional losses of water through urine and sweat. One should take the opportunity to ingest carbohydrates, about 50 g of glucose on average within the first two hours after the exercise, for re-synthesis of muscular glucogen to take place, along with a swift storage of muscular and hepatic glycogen (McArdle et al. 2001; Wilmore and Costill, 2004).

Condition	% Body weight change	Urine colour	Urine specific gravity
Well hydrated	+1 to –1	1 or 2	< 1.010
Minimal dehydration	–1 to –3	3 or 4	1.010 – 1.020
Significant dehydration	–3 –5	5 or 6	1.021 – 1.030
Serious dehydration	> 5	> 6	> 1.030

MONITORING

It is important that athletes monitor their own hydration status. They should be aware of the symptoms of dehydration, of how to use urine volume and colour as an indicator of hydration status and the importance of pre and post body weight measurements.

Table Indices of Hydration Status (general guidelines)

Signs and symptoms of dehydration include thirst, irritability, and general discomfort, followed by headache, weakness, dizziness, cramps, chills, vomiting, nausea, head or neck heat sensations and decreased performance.

Thirst is a poor indicator of the need to drink to drink. Thirst indicates that 1.5-2.0l fluid have already been lost.

References

Bodil Nielsen,Gisela Sjogaard G,J Udelvig,Bo Knudsen and B Dohlmanna 1986,Fluid balanc in exercise dehydration and rehydration with different glucose electrolyte drinks, *European journal of Applied physiology*; 55(3), 318-325.

Byrne C, Lim CL, Chew SA, Ming ET. Water versus carbohydrate-electrolyte fluid replacement during loaded marching under heat stress. Mil Med. 2005; 170: 715-21.

Fallowfield JL, Williams C, Singh R. The influence of ingesting a carbohydrate-electrolyte beverage during 4 hours of recovery on subsequent endurance capacity. *Int J Sports Nutr* 1995; 5: 285-99.

Guyton AC and Hall JE. Textbook of Medical Physiology. W.B. Saunders Company; NY, 10th ed, 2000.

Jung AP, Bishop PA, Al-Nawwas A, Dale RB. Influence of Hydration and Electrolyte Supplementation on Incidence and Time to Onset of Exercise-Associated Muscle Cramps. J Athl Train. 2005; 40: 71-75.

Khanna GL, Manna I. Supplementary effect of carbohydrate-electrolyte drink on sports performance, lactate removal & cardiovascular response of athletes. Indian J Med Res. 2005; 121: 665-9.

Maughan RJ, Shirreffs SM, Watson P. Exercise, heat, hydration and the brain. J Am Coll Nutr. 2007 26: 604S-612S.

McArdle WD et al. Exercise Physiology: Energy, Nutrition, and Human Performance. Lippincott Williams & Wilkins; NY, 5 ed, 2001.

Mohamed Saat, Rabindarjeet Singh, Roland Gamini Sirisinghe and Mohd Nawawi, Rehydration after Exercise with Fresh Young Coconut Water, carbohydrate-Electrolyte Beverage and Plain Water, *Journal of PHYSIOLOGICAL ANTHROPOLOGY and Applied Human Science* 21. 2002, 93-104

Montain SJ, Cheuvront SN, Sawka MN. Exercise associated hyponatraemia: quantitative analysis to understand the aetiology. Br J Sports Med. 2006; 40: 98-105; discussion 98-105.

Nicholas CW, Williams C, Lakomy HKA, Phillips G, Nowitz A. Influence of ingesting a carbohydrate-electrolyte solution on endurance capacity during intermittent highintensity shuttle running. *J Sports Sci* 1995; 13: 283-90.

Oppliger RA, Magnes SA, Popowski LA, Gisolfi CV.Accuracy of urine specific gravity and osmolality as indicators of hydration status.Int J Sport Nutr Exerc Metab. 2005; 15: 236-51.

Rehrer NJ. Fluid and electrolyte balance in ultra-endurance sport. Sports Med. 2001; 31(10): 701-15.

Sawka MN, Burke LM, Eichner ER, Maughan RJ, Montain SJ, Stachenfeld NS. American College of Sports Medicine position stand. Exercise and fluid replacement. Med Sci Sports Exerc. 2007; 39: 377-90.

Shirreffs SM, Aragon-Vargas LF, Keil M, Love TD, Phillips S. Rehydration after exercise in the heat: a comparison of 4 commonly used drinks. Int J Sport Nutr Exerc Metab. 2007; 17: 244-58.

Shirreffs SM, Maughan RJ. The effect of alcohol on athletic performance. Curr Sports Med Rep. 2006; 5: 192-6.

Tsintzas OK, Williams C, Boobis L, Greenhaff P. Carbohydrate ingestion and single muscle fiber glycogen metabolism during prolonged running in men. *J Appl Physiol* 1996b *81*: 801-9.

Tsintzas OK, Williams C, Wilson W, Burrin J. Influence of carbohydrate supplementation early in exercise on endurance running capacity. *Med Sci Sports Exerc* 1996a *28*: 1373-9.

Wilmore JH and Costill D. L. Physiology of Sport and Exercise. Human Kinetics Publishers; NY, 3Rev Ed, 2004.